英文医学科研论文 写作与发表

朱冰倩◎主编

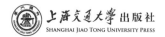
上海交通大学出版社
SHANGHAI JIAO TONG UNIVERSITY PRESS

内容提要

本书基于开展医学科学研究的基本过程，系统地介绍了医学科研论文常见范式和论文发表流程。全书共 8 章。第 1 章，概述撰写科研论文的重要性、必要性和可行性，并对常见科研论文类型进行总结，为后续章节奠定理论基础。第 2～5 章，分别对不同类型医学科研论文的撰写要点进行深入剖析（包括系统文献综述和原创性论著，如临床研究论文、基础研究论文、质性研究论文），为读者提供基本思路。第 6 章，着重介绍撰写英文医学科研论文时常用的格式，提醒读者需要注意的细节性错误。第 7 章，详细介绍投稿和发表流程，指导读者选择合适的期刊并顺利完成投稿、修回和发表。第 8 章，总结撰写和发表科研论文过程中涉及的伦理和学术规范，进而培养读者严谨的科研态度。

本书可作为医学生论文写作课程的辅助教材，也可作为科研人员学术研究素养的参考读物。

图书在版编目(CIP)数据

英文医学科研论文：写作与发表/朱冰倩主编. —
上海：上海交通大学出版社，2022.5
ISBN 978 - 7 - 313 - 26803 - 7

Ⅰ.①英...　Ⅱ.①朱...　Ⅲ.①医学－英语－论文－写作　Ⅳ.①R

中国版本图书馆 CIP 数据核字(2022)第 073593 号

英文医学科研论文——写作与发表
YINGWEN YIXUE KEYAN LUNWEN —— XIEZUO YU FABIAO

主　　编：朱冰倩			
出版发行：上海交通大学出版社		地　　址：上海市番禺路 951 号
邮政编码：200030		电　　话：021 - 64071208
印　　制：上海盛通时代印刷有限公司		经　　销：全国新华书店
开　　本：880mm×1230mm　1/32		印　　张：8.25
字　　数：212 千字		
版　　次：2022 年 5 月第 1 版		印　　次：2022 年 5 月第 1 次印刷
书　　号：ISBN 978 - 7 - 313 - 26803 - 7		
定　　价：50.00 元		

编委会名单

主　编　朱冰倩
副主编　林可可　郭　蕾
编　委（按姓氏笔画排序）
　　　　于明明　北京大学护理学院
　　　　石长贵　海军军医大学第二附属医院（上海长征医院）
　　　　朱冰倩　上海交通大学护理学院
　　　　张婧珺　西安交通大学护理系
　　　　林可可　北京中医药大学护理学院
　　　　郭　蕾　上海交通大学医学院

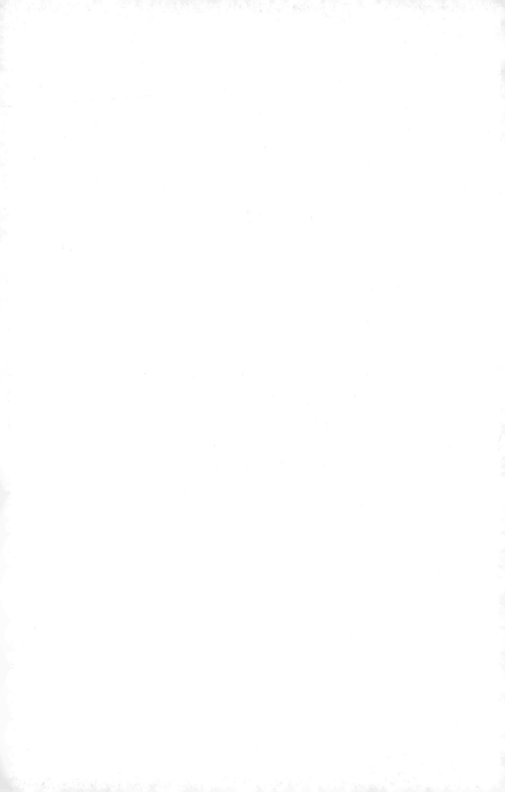

前　言

I was taught that the way of progress was neither swift nor easy

——居里夫人

　　撰写及发表科研论文是科学研究中一个不可缺少的核心环节。目前,多数高校均要求研究生在毕业之前,能够在相关学科期刊上发表科研论文。因此,亟需一些指导性强、实用度高、覆盖面广的书籍,帮助学生及科研人员掌握撰写和发表期刊论文的技能。本书的编写立足国际前沿、以高质量教学为指导,以科研能力提升为导向,具有先进性、科学性和实用性。

　　不同于既往书籍,本书具有以下特色:

　　1. 立足国际,前沿性好

　　本书编写团队由专职科研人员和教师构成,团队成员均具有海外留学背景(主编为美国留学博士),具有丰富的科研论文撰写和发表经历。在撰写过程中,团队成员不仅立足国际前沿、充分运用常年积累的撰写经验,更是融入审稿过程中的心得体会。因此,本书在团队上具有创新性和先进性。

　　2. 引用典范,实用性强

　　本书以发表在不同领域高水平期刊的论文为典范,通过对其进行剖析,为读者提供标准化、高水平的论文撰写和发表建议。书中涉及的案例均来自编写成员的亲身经历,为读者规避撰写科研论文中常见的错误提供了实用建议。读者可结合自己的经历，将理论技能应用到实践中。因此，本书在内容上具有准确性和实用性。

3. 言简意赅、趣味性足

本书简洁明了地凝练了学生需要掌握的论文撰写和发表要点。在书中，减少了冗长枯燥的文字描述，通过运用现实案例，增强学生的阅读兴趣。因此，本书在形式上具有多样性和趣味性。

4. 基于需求、辐射面广

本书的撰写基于广大医学生及科研人员的需求，着重介绍英文医学科研论文的撰写和发表。本书的适用对象包括"对撰写科研论文毫无头绪"的本科生、研究生和"为撰写科研论文而苦恼"的科研人员（包括博士后及青年教师），适用于临床医学、护理学、公共卫生、预防医学、基础医学等专业。因此，本书在服务上具有针对性和广泛性。

本书共8章，涵盖了医学科研论文中的常见类型。对于未涉及的其他类型论文，可在参考本书的基础上进行相应的调整。书末附有参考文献，以便读者进行更加深入的阅读和学习。本书将为成功发表英文医学科研论文提供以下独特的知识和技能：

（1）以理论原则为指导，从实践角度出发，具体介绍"如何去做"。

（2）通过举例，详细说明撰写和发表不同类型科研论文的实用方法。

（3）针对写作和发表过程中"该做什么"和"不该做什么"给出建议。

（4）针对常用汇报指南或清单，提供重要、实用的网络资源（网站）。

此次写作之旅充满了挑战，但是很幸运在此过程中遇到了优秀的同事、朋友和学生。因此，要特别感谢她们在此过程中提供的帮助和指导。首先，十分感谢本书的编委在繁忙工作之余，仍旧抽出时间参与各章节的编撰,毫无保留地分享自己的经验、贡献自己的智慧。其次,感谢上海交通大学护理学院朱大乔教授在前期准备工作中提供的鼓励以及在本书编撰过程中提供的宝贵建议;感谢我的研究生陈沛、王月莹、牟云平及袁金金在书稿校对过程中提供的帮助。再者,感谢以下同事和朋友在用户调研方面提供的信息和数据:吴映晖(上海交通大学)、程丽副教授(中山大学)、颜萍教授(新疆医科大学)、王涛副教授(海南医学院)。最后,感谢上海交通大学出版社整个编辑出版团队为本书的出版提供平台、为本书封面的设计及内容的校对提供支持。

朱冰倩

2022 年 4 月

目　录

第❶章 绪 论

　　科学研究的开展是一个严谨而复杂的循环过程，在此过程中，科研论文的撰写和发表是推动科学进步不可或缺的重要环节。科研论文的撰写对于科研人员的文献阅读和整合能力及逻辑性和评判性思维都具有很高的要求。然而，科研论文的撰写并不是无章可循，它是一个有着规范性、严谨性和可复制性的科学活动。本章中，我们将回答以下几个问题。

- 科学研究包括哪几个环节？
- 为何要撰写和发表科研论文？
- 撰写论文有哪些常见障碍及如何克服？
- 常见论文类型及撰写论文需要做哪些准备工作？

第1节 科学研究过程

　　科学研究是通过运用科学方法和科学原理揭示不同变量之间的关系，以找出解决问题的方案或发展新的理论，多由科研人员通过系统的方法学实现。根据现有的理论，一个完整的科研周期，大致包括5个环节，如图1-1所示。这5个环节呈非线性循序渐进，形成一个闭环，可以重复开展。

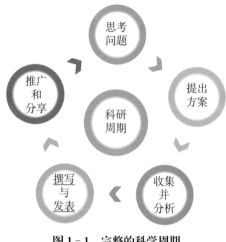

图 1 - 1　完整的科学周期

环节一：思考问题

　　思考并发现研究问题是科学研究活动的第一步，也是最重要的一步。这一阶段处于科研活动的准备阶段，研究人员根据自己的实践经验、结合日常观察和好奇心、通过阅读文献等途径对相关问题进行头脑风暴，经过反复的思考和总结，最终形成科研问题。

环节二：提出方案

　　针对科研问题，提出相应的计划方案是开展科学研究的第二个环节。此阶段中，科研人员从战略上提出科学、可靠、可行的实施方案，进而回答第一阶段提出的科研问题。为了高效地实施此阶段科研活动，科研人员可创建一个信息存储系统，将获取的信息围绕关键主题进行分类存储。成熟、严谨的研究方案，对于开展下一环节的科研活动至关重要。

环节三：收集并分析

科研活动的第三个环节是,根据环节二提出的方案,进行数据收集和分析。围绕研究问题,对所收集的数据进行系统化分类、整理和筛选。根据研究问题不同,采用不同的方法对数据进行分析和整合。

环节四：撰写与发表

科研活动的第四个环节是,撰写并发表科研论文。通过此阶段科研活动,将研究结果发表在学术期刊上,以促进科研人员之间的对话和交流;同时又为下一步研究提出启发和指导。**这也是本书的介绍重点。**

环节五：推广和分享

除了通过论文的形式,还可通过其他形式对研究成果进行推广和分享。常见的途径包括:参加国内外学术会议、在科研组会/研讨会中进行分享、在学术委员会议中进行分享等。通过将相应的研究发现与前辈、同辈、同行及其他领域的专家及大众进行分享,扩大研究成果的辐射面。此环节科研活动还可为发现新的科研问题提供思路。

第2节　科研论文撰写与发表

与开展科学研究类似,论文发表也是一个包含多个环节、具有反复性的过程,如**图 1-2** 所示。"论文创作"环节中,形成论文初稿。

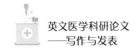
紧接着,进入"论文评价",通过接受同事或同行的反馈意见或评价,不断提高论文质量。"论文发表"环节中,涉及出版商对论文的格式、布局等进行编辑,并提供出版服务。已经发表的论文将进入"传播获取"环节,此环节中,论文通过图书馆、网页等途径,以纸质或电子版本的形式在读者中进行传播、扩散。最后,"论文使用"环节中,论文得到阅读、引用和整合。**本书将着重对"发表周期"中的论文创作和发表进行详细介绍。**

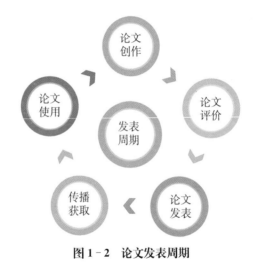

图 1‑2　论文发表周期

　　许多读者常常会有这样一个疑问:为什么要撰写和发表科研论文?不将研究成果发表出去,类似于制造了某个产品,而不将其发布出来。发表科研论文对作者本人、他人、学科及社会发展均具有必要性和重要性。

1. 作者本人

　　(1)发表科研论文是科研工作者不可或缺的一个能力:如前所

述,发表论文是科学研究中一个重要环节,对于想要从事科研工作的人来说,撰写和发表科研论文的能力不足将大大阻碍其在科研道路上的成长。

(2) 发表科研论文有利于增加知识储备、跟进最新研究进展: 在撰写和发表科研论文过程中,作者本人需要对现有文献进行回顾,并将最新研究发现与自己的研究进行对比分析。这将有助于扩展个人知识储备,并与现阶段研究保持同步。

(3) 发表科研论文可促进职业发展: 论文发表是评价一个人科研能力的重要指标,许多高校和科研机构鼓励开展科研工作,这些工作可以促进新知识的产生并带来创新。目前,论文发表情况是许多用人单位对个人进行考核的指标之一,发表论文有利于个人职业发展。

(4) 发表科研论文可提高个人在相关研究领域的知名度: 如果个体针对某特定主题或问题发表了大量的科研论文,其将获得较高的信誉并成为该领域公认的专家。此知名度会使得个人在为单位、政府和非政府机构建言资政时,具有一定的话语权。

(5) 发表科研论文有助于提升个人的满足感和成就感: 科研写作是一个烦琐、漫长的过程。经过此过程后,成功发表论文既是对个人付出的回报,也是对其能力的肯定;这可以大大增进其信心以及满足感和成就感。

2. 他人

(1) 为他人开展科研提供思路和启发: 科研论文发表后,研究成果会在全球各地进行扩散,这为与他人进行知识和证据分享以及经验交流提供了机会。同时,他人通过阅读你的研究成果,可以有效避免重复性科研工作,有助于加快科研进展。

(2) 为开展科研合作提供机会: 科学无地域和国界,他人读到你

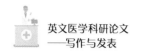
的研究成果后,可能会寻求你的专业帮助和建议;这也可为你们今后开展科研合作提供契机。

(3)激发热情、激励研究:你的科研可能会激发许多学生和科研人员对于该领域的兴趣和热情;你的研究结果也可能激励许多开展类似研究的科研人员不断坚持和创新。

3. 学科

(1)提升专业信誉和知名度:科研人员通过运用高质量的研究证据,提高临床实践、指导政策制定,进而推动人类健康水平的提升。在此过程中,社会大众对于该学科的认识度也会得到提升。因此,论文发表对于提升专业信誉和知名度也具有重要意义。

(2)充实学科知识体系:科学研究是一个学科发展的重要基石,新的科研发现将丰富某特定主题的知识库。这些研究发现可能会支持有些学者的论点,而反驳了另一些学者的论点,这将激发科研人员开展进一步研究去阐明科学问题,建立和完善相关理论,进而充实学科知识体系。当然,某一学科知识体系的完善,也将从广义上推动知识积累和科学发展。

4. 社会发展

(1)完善已有实践标准,促进人类健康:随着科学的进步、新的研究工具的出现,以前被广泛遵循的实践标准也许不再科学和实用。通过结合最新研究成果,临床工作人员可以批判性地反思已有的临床实践标准,进而对其进行修订和完善。高质量的研究成果可以指导临床实践、提高医疗服务质量,最终促进人类健康并推动社会发展。

(2)通过参与政策制定,推动社会进步:研究结果对政策制定非常重要,基于科学证据的政策可以节省大量时间、金钱和精力,避免不必要的错误和资源浪费。如果决策者了解最新科学研究进展,则可制定出更加科学的政策。在许多发达国家,科研人员是政府和非政府机构决策中的重要参与者。从此方面来看,科研成果可以推动社会发展和进步。

第3节　撰写科研论文常见障碍及应对策略

撰写医学科研论文具有很大的挑战性,而英文与中文论文的撰写更存在天壤之别,不仅是在写作风格上,更体现在语言的应用上。撰写和发表英文科研论文过程中,常见的障碍和挑战大致可归纳为4个方面。

1. 常见障碍

(1) **缺少时间**。没有(成块的)时间,始终是多数人认为的主要障碍。科研写作需要投入大量的时间和精力,随着科研人员职业生涯的发展,其可自由调配的时间变得越来越少;科技进步和电子产品的广泛使用也常常干扰人们的工作进程和效率。因此,能够全身心投入写作的时间也会大大减少。但是,仍有很多人可以完成大量的科研论文,而且他们似乎并没有比其他人花费更多的时间。那么,他们是如何做到的? 接下来,本书将会进行解答。

(2) **害怕论文被拒**。害怕论文被拒是许多学者面临的一个心理挑战。论文被拒会使个人的信心受挫,它会给人一种错觉:让人以为被拒的不仅仅是论文,还有论文写作者这个"人"。从无到有的突破往往最具挑战性。因此,成功发表第一篇论文对于克服害怕被拒这种心理负担十分重要。而想要成功发表,掌握核心写作技巧则是

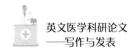

必备条件。

(3) 科研写作能力不足，未能掌握核心技巧。 写作能力不足是撰写科研论文中面临的一个主要障碍，有时候，这种不足甚至会演变成写作者的一种恐惧。这种恐惧源于缺乏实战经验和机会，更可惜的是，也可能源于既往的不良经历（例如，写作早期遭到老师、同学、同事等的轻视）。有这种写作恐惧的人可能为了待在自己的舒适圈，乐于抛弃写作，直到由于毕业或者工作所需，才重新开始继续写作。此外，写作和发表过程中还会涉及许多技巧（例如，针对不同的读者，对论文背景等应进行相应调整）。未能掌握这些核心技巧，也是影响开展有效科研写作的一个主要障碍。

(4) 不了解发表过程。 任何新鲜事物的学习都是一个充满挑战的过程。论文发表涉及一个漫长的周期，短则两三个月（虽然不常见），长则一年多。发表过程本身涵盖多个步骤：从选择合适的期刊、准备投稿清单、投稿，到论文修回，再到校样的审阅。这些过程，对于很多人来说都是陌生的领域。因此，对科研论文发表过程的不了解有可能成为快速、有效发表的一个障碍。

2. 应对策略

当然，任何问题都有对策或解决方法。面对上述常见障碍，在使用此书的时候，建议结合以下三大策略进行有效应对。

(1) 建立写作计划，进行有效时间管理。 在学习和工作的长期计划中，纳入"撰写和发表论文"，根据自己的实际情况制订计划。例如：每年在同行评审的国际期刊上发表至少一篇论文。一旦确定了长期计划，需要进一步明确每周（或每个工作日）的写作计划。每天要完成的写作不需要很多（例如，一段文字），但是贵在坚持。这样的习惯可以保证你在完成其他任务的同时（例如，学习、实习、工作），一直都可以沉浸在写作过程中，保证连贯性。根据个人情况，制订合理、可行的写作目标或字数目标。例如,我在创作此章节时,设定的目标是1~1.5页/天(1500~2000字)。有些学者建议,完成目标后就停止当日写作,因为有时候试图完成更多任务,效果往往会适得其反。当然,还有一种策略是:使用小标题记录下后面一天需要完成的写作内容。此策略既可以帮助你及时记录下当下的写作灵感,也有利于第二天快速进入写作状态(仅需要根据列好的小标题进行扩展)。多数期刊论文是有字数要求的,在写作过程中需要通过数字数了解自己的写作进展。数字数也是一个正反馈,可以激励你继续写作。当然,每个人都会出现写作思路被困的时候(不知道该写什么),此时就很容易放弃当天的写作计划。但是,建议你开始写下一部分内容,或回头看看写过的东西里是否需要添加其他内容,直到完成今日的写作目标。你可以修改写得不好的地方,但是无法对空白页进行编辑。只要有了任何写作灵感,就应该立马把它记下来。为了进行有效的时间管理,需要预留出专门的写作时间,进而完成每天的写作任务。当然,这并不是要求每天投入半天甚至全天于写作中。可以仅在工作效率最高的时候,抽出1~2个小时(甚至半个小时)用于写作。充分利用好片段时间,对于坚持写作十分重要。

(2) **把论文"被拒"当成进一步完善作品的宝贵机会。**论文被拒是每个学者都面临过的问题(即使是学术权威),也是论文发表过程中的重要组成部分(尤其对于学术期刊)。有时候,论文被拒反而是一件好事。因为这些审稿人或编辑多是熟悉你的研究领域并具有一定国际学术声誉的专家,你可以从他们那里免费获取非常宝贵的反馈意见。你可以根据这些建议,进一步完善论文,为下一次投稿做好准备。当然,了解被拒稿的原因可以有助于下一次投稿。本书会在后面的章节中进行详细介绍。

(3) **积极寻求反馈和评判。**撰写完第一稿后,就要开始修改论文。最有经验的作家也很少会在第一次就呈现出最好的作品,对于科研写作更是如此。写作经验越丰富,后期需要投入修改的时间和精力就会越少。具体如何修改论文,后面的章节中会详细介绍。多数情况下,修改完初稿后,先将其搁置几天,然后再重新返回进行修改,这种时间差会帮助你拥有不同的视角。一旦你对自己改好的文字比较满意了,就可以将其发送给老师或同事等进行阅读,寻求他们的意见和建议。保持一种开放心态,积极寻求他人反馈是一种严谨的科研态度,也是科学工作者应具备的基本品质。寻求别人的意见绝非易事,人们往往会担心其他人对自己的工作给出负面评论。但是,以下建议会使你在接受他人评论的时候,觉得更轻松:①越是寻求批评,就越容易接受批评,也越容易成为更好的学者和作家。②你是在为别人写作,并不是在为自己而写作。因此,其他人(潜在的读者)是你写作的最佳裁判。③别人给出的评论是针对你的论文,并不是针对你个人。因此,一旦完成了初稿,建议找 1~2 个人进行审阅,为你提供意见。最好是 2 个人,这样获取的反馈会更加全面,同时也避免了人数太多而造成评论"轰炸"。在反馈意见方面,论文发表经验丰富的同事和经验不足的同事对你都是有益的。有经验的同事多可以对论文总体结构和论点质量给出建议,此外,他们可能了解某些编辑和期刊的偏好,这将对你大有裨益。经验不足的同事或者与你的研究领域相关度不大的学者,经常会询问"这是什么意思?"或指出"这没有道理",以局外人的视角,为你提供宝贵建议。

在科研论文写作过程中,必须要学会接受批评。如果负面反馈可以帮助提高论文质量,那么它们带来的效果就是正面的。如果在投稿之前,没有收到适当的反馈,你或许将从期刊编辑和审稿人那里得到批评,结果可能会更严重,常常会导致论文被拒(论文写作质量差是被拒的最常见原因之一)。需要指出的是,你要向信任的人寻求反馈,不要向总是消极、给出负反馈的人寻求意见,因为他们的建议可能是破坏性而非建设性的。类似地,也不要向害怕给别人提建议的人寻求反馈,因为你无法从他们那里获取任何建设性建议。

良好的写作习惯是完成科研论文的基础,掌握核心技巧是写好科研论文的必备条件。本书在剩余的章节中，将着重介绍如何有效应对"写作能力不足，未能掌握核心技巧"及"不了解发表过程"。

第4节　常见论文类型及撰写论文准备工作

科研论文中比较常见的类型是论著（article）。对于论著，根据论文是否基于研究过程中收集到的一手数据，可以分为原创性论著（original article）或综述（review article）。根据研究问题以及学科不同，原创性论著可大致分为三大类：临床研究论文、基础研究论文和质性研究论文。除此之外，常见的论文形式还包括：病例报告（case report）、社论（editorial）、述评（comment）、读者来信（letter）等。对于论著，虽然不同类型的论著书写格式和重点有所差异，但这几种论文的撰写都有共通之处。因此，在对这几种类型论文的撰写要点进行详细介绍之前，先对其通用原则进行简要概述。

1. 开始写作前，需要完成的准备工作

（1）明确论文所要传达的信息及目标读者：在开始撰写论文前，最好先明确论文想要传达的信息及潜在读者群，此准备工作可大大推动后期写作进程。当然，有些学者习惯在后期修改过程中，针对读者群对论文内容进行相应的调整。对于论文想要传达的信息，切忌内容太多。例如，很难在一篇论文中体现出来博士课题所完成的所有研究内容。此时，就需要对一个大的科研项目进行分割，在一篇论文中回答某一个明确的研究问题。同时，也要避免撰写"香肠论文"（salami publication），即为了增加所发表论文的数量，将数据进行不合理切割（详见第8章）。对于目标读者，选择合适的期刊很重要，可以通过仔细阅读目标期刊的目的和范围（aim and scope）来确定。后

续章节中,会对如何选择期刊展开详细介绍。虽然无法确定论文一定会被某个期刊接收,但是在撰写论文前或过程中,确定一个目标期刊(target journal)对于指导写作是有帮助的。选定目标期刊,可以帮助你适当地关注此期刊一般都发表什么样的论文以及你的论文与此期刊的契合度。

选择期刊时,有人主张首先从你感兴趣的领域中按照其受欢迎度(或影响因子)开始,由高到低依次尝试,直到稿件被接收。有时候,你可能很幸运,稿件被接收。但是,你必须要知道:期刊越有声望,被拒绝的可能性就越大。当然,对于质量很高(在某领域发现重大突破)的论文,可以尝试此种方法。值得注意的是,一篇论文是否适合某期刊,主要是看这篇论文是否适合该期刊的读者,而不是根据影响因子。有经验的作者也许能够更好地判断他们的论文投到哪里更容易被接收。后文中,会详细介绍如何选择合适的目标期刊。

(2)仔细阅读投稿指南(author guidelines): 从目标期刊的网站上寻找投稿指南,仔细阅读每一条指南。

● **期刊接收论文的形式:** 首先,通过阅读投稿指南,确定期刊接收论文的类型。常见论文类型包括:原创性论著、综述、个案报道等。值得注意的是,有些期刊不接收综述类论文或仅约稿综述。明确期刊接收论文的类型,对于指导后期撰写也具有一定作用。

● **确定目标期刊所接收论文的最大字数(word limit)。** 通常情况下,原创性论著和综述的字数限制有所不同(例如,原创性论著正文多不超过5 000字,而综述正文多不超过8 000字)。某些期刊允许:在与编辑协商解释后,可以超过字数限制。这种情况常常发生于综述中,因为综述常包含对于多个论文的回顾和分析,作者需要详细描述检索过程,对论文之间的差异进行解释。了解期刊的字数限制,你在撰写论文过程中心里就有了一杆秤。当然,论文也不能太短,否则无法向读者阐明重要的研究细节,而使得审稿人无法全面地对你的论文进行评审。

- 熟悉目标期刊对论文组织构架的要求。投稿指南中,通常会说明论文需要包含的标题和子标题。为进一步明确,可以下载该期刊最近发表的论文,参考其撰写结构。原创性论著和系统综述在组织结构上可能存在一定的差异,注意区分。论文的组织结构非常重要,它为论文提供了方向,可有利于读者快速地定位到自己感兴趣的位置。多数读者并不会完全读完一篇论文,只是挑选自己感兴趣的地方,比如研究涉及领域、统计分析方法、结果。因此,在准备期间,应该明确期刊对于论文结构的要求;在撰写期间,应确保在适当的标题下提供相应的内容。当然,有些期刊对标题没有特殊要求,这个时候,可以参考自己的研究领域常见期刊的组织构架形式。

- **论文布局**:注意字体、字号、行间距等细节;按照期刊要求进行书写,使得编辑读起来一目了然,给他们留下深刻的第一印象。期刊编辑都很繁忙,并没有时间帮你去完成格式等方面的修改。根据一些国际高水平期刊编辑的反馈:如果收到的稿件没有按照期刊的要求格式进行撰写,幸运的话,稿件会被退回,期刊接受修改后再投;不幸运的话,直接在送外审之前就被拒稿,尤其是针对一些创新性和特色不是很突出的稿件。对于英语非母语的中国学者而言,语法的规范和准确性也是一个值得注意的地方。目前,很多润色公司可以提供语言润色等服务。但是,多数润色公司仅提供语法上的修改,往往无法针对论文的逻辑性和相关性进行修改。这时如果向英语为母语或在英文论文撰写方面比较有经验的学者寻求反馈意见,不失为一种有效方法。因为他们不仅可以提供语言上的帮助,还能够针对论文的内容提供修改建议。

- **论文汇报指南(reporting guidelines)**:目前,越来越多的期刊都要求论文的汇报参照特定的指南。其目的主要是通过促进研究报告的透明度和准确性来提高卫生健康相关文献的可靠性和价值。**常见的指南包括:CONSORT**(针对随机试验)、**STROBE**(针对观察性研究)和 **PRISMA**(针对系统综述)。对于临床试验,一般在汇报时,需

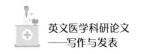

要提供研究注册号;对于文献综述,有些期刊要求提供综述方案注册号(例如,PROSPERO)。对于所有报告,都有说明研究是否通过伦理审查以及相对应的审查机构。这方面的具体内容将会在后面详细介绍。以下网站中,罗列了不同类型论文的汇报指南:https://www.equator-network.org/。

● **审稿费和版面费**:多数期刊不需要审稿费,但个别期刊会有一定的审稿费(例如,50 美元)。不论稿件是否被接受,审稿费都不予退回。有些期刊对于接收的论文还会提供开放获取(open access)这一选项,收取一定的版面费。在投稿之前,需要看清楚该期刊是不是仅刊出 open access 论文。有些期刊,虽然一般情况下不收取版面费,但对于彩图是需要收取费用的,在投稿前也需进行了解。

2. 确定撰写提纲

一般情况下,论著的撰写提纲包括:标题(Title)、摘要(Abstract)、前言或背景(Introduction/Background)、方法或材料(Methods/Materials)、结果(Results)、讨论(Discussion)、结论(Conclusion)、参考文献(References)、图表(Tables and Figures)。接下来的各个章节中,将详细介绍每一部分内容如何书写。

第 ② 章　原创性论著撰写要点

——临床研究论文

在循证医学的指导下,越来越多的医疗决策依赖于严谨、科学的临床研究证据,撰写和发表临床论文则成为促进临床实践不可缺少的一部分。本章对临床论文的撰写要点进行详细介绍,通过引用多个案例,深入浅出地讲解完成一篇临床论文的撰写要点。本章中,我们将回答以下几个问题。

- 如何撰写言简意赅、有吸引力的标题、摘要和关键词?
- 如何构建简洁明了、有逻辑性的前言和(或)背景?
- 什么是研究方法的八股文撰写法?
- 如何合理地呈现主要研究结果?
- 如何撰写一个完整、具有层次感的讨论?
- 如何合理分配一篇论文各个部分的篇幅?
- 汇报临床论文,可参考哪些汇报指南?

第1节　标题和摘要

1. 标题

标题(Title)十分重要,应尽可能言简意赅。许多人阅读文献时，首先读的是标题。一个好标题能激发读者的兴趣，也能帮助读者快速、准确地检索到你的论文。有时候，审稿人可能会建议你更改标题，尤其是当他们认为论文标题不能很好地反映论文内容的时候。另外一些时候，编辑会根据自己的期刊对于标题的要求，对你的论文标题进行修改，以增加论文的"可发现性"（discoverability）。

一般情况下，论文的标题需要包括研究涉及的重要信息，例如**研究内容、人群和设计**。多数期刊要求：标题中首先要体现主要研究内容，然后，使用"**冒号**"，紧接着给出研究设计，例如：Cognitive behavioral therapy in the treatment of insomnia: A randomized clinical trial。目前，还有一种趋势：**把最重要**的信息最早呈现在标题中。此时，使用以下标题就更合适：A randomized clinical trial of cognitive behavioral therapy in the treatment of insomnia。

当然，还有一些标题没有体现研究设计，而是体现了研究在**数据收集或统计分析**方面的特色。例如：Depression and self-care in older adults with multiple chronic conditions: A multivariate analysis.

类似地，还有一些标题仅描述了研究主要内容和人群。例如：Development and validation of a Clinical Risk Score to predict the occurrence of critical illness in hospitalized patients with COVID-19。

还有些标题开门见山，在标题中体现**研究的主要发现**，例如：Mild to moderate partial sleep deprivation is associated with increased impulsivity and decreased positive affect in young adults.

虽然不常见，但有些标题采用了提问的形式。例如：Are there differences in pain intensity between two consecutive vaginal childbirths? A retrospective cohort study.

以上的示例中，不管采用了何种形式，最主要的特点就是言简意赅、内容翔实且有吸引力。另外，有些期刊对于标题的字数有限制。在投稿前，应进行核查。此外，还可下载目标期刊最近发表的论文，对比一下自己的标题和它们所接收论文的标题在格式上是否一致。

撰写标题时，除了以上在内容上需要遵循的原则，在格式上也需要注意：

（1）有些期刊要求标题中的单词书写须使用首字母大写（title case），具体规则如下。

以下情况，首字母须大写：

- 标题（及副标题）的第一个单词（即使这个单词是虚词）。
- 位于冒号、破折号、点号后面的第一个单词（即使这个单词是虚词）。
- 所有实词（包括名词、动词、形容词、数词、量词及代词），包括连字符后面那个单词的首字母（例如，Self-Report）。
- 包含 4 个及以上字母的虚词（例如，With，Among，Between，From）。
- 专有名词或量表中的各个单词。

以下情况，使用小写：

- 所有含有 **3 个及以下**字母的虚词，包括连词（例如，and，as，but）、介词（例如，as，via，by）和冠词（例如，a，an，the）。

具体例子，如下：The Association Between Self-Report Sleep and Cognitive Function in Older Adults：A Multilevel Analysis

（2）许多期刊要求标题中的单词使用句首大写（sentence case），具体规则如下。

- 标题（及副标题）的第一个单词首字母须大写（即使这个单词是虚词）。
- 位于冒号、破折号、点号后面的第一个单词首字母须大写（即使这个单词是虚词）。

- 专有名词或量表中各个单词的首字母须大写。
- 其他单词均使用小写。

具体例子,如下:The association between sleep measured by Insomnia Severity Index and cognitive function in older adults:A multilevel analysis。

(3) 避免在标题中使用缩写(除非该缩写很常见且不使用缩写的情况下,标题字数会超过期刊要求,例如,HIV)。

2. 摘要

(1) **摘要的重要性。** 摘要的重要性不言而喻。许多读者仅阅读一篇论文的摘要,而不会花大量的时间阅读全文。因此,摘要中要展现论文的精华部分。这个对于其他学者进行论文检索尤为重要。例如,在进行系统综述时,其中一个步骤是对所检索到的论文进行筛查,初筛阶段仅阅读标题和摘要,如果摘要不够全面,那么你的论文就会被漏掉,减少其被引用的概率。更重要的是,稿件提交后第一个阅读(审阅)它的人就是编辑。如果摘要不够清晰、规范,那么稿件很可能在送外审之前就被拒。编辑可能认为:既然摘要都不符合规范,那么正文可能也没有按照投稿指南书写。因此,摘要呈现给编辑的第一印象非常重要。

(2) **摘要的基本要求。** 同标题一样,摘要内容需要简短而丰富。一般情况下,字数在200~300字(具体因期刊而异)。避免在摘要中使用引文,有的期刊甚至要求摘要中不能包含缩写。为了更好地呈现,本书较早地介绍了摘要的书写要求。但一般情况下,摘要会留到全文完成后再写。

(3) **摘要的格式。** 一般情况下,摘要的格式可分为**结构式和非结构式**。无论是哪种形式,均需要使读者读完以后,知道你的研究做了什么? 怎么做? 发现了什么? 研究发现有何启示? **结构式摘要需**

要给出小标题,包括：背景/目的,方法,结果和结论。根据期刊不同,"背景"可能不需要。有的期刊要求在介绍"方法"前面,有个单独的标题"设计(Design)"(具体格式需要参照相应的期刊进行完善)。对于**非结构式**摘要,虽然它不要求给出小标题,但是需要包括上述提到的各部分内容。接下来,将对已发表论文的摘要进行剖析,进一步说明每个部分的撰写要点。

1) 结构式摘要。

① **研究目的(Aim,Purpose 或 Objective)。**"研究目的"这一部分,有些杂志在"投稿指南"里指明,直接给出"To examine..."。此时,作者就开门见山:To examine...。如示例 2 - 1 和示例 2 - 2 所示。示例 2 - 1 中,作者还在摘要中给出了研究假设(hypothesis)。

示例 2 - 1　研究目的举例 1

Study objectives：To examine the association between duration trajectories over 28 years and measures of cognition, gray matter volume, and white matter microstructure. We hypothesize that consistently meeting sleep guidelines that recommend at least 7 hours of sleep per night will be associated with better cognition, greater gray matter volumes, higher fractional anisotropy, and lower radial diffusivity values.

示例 2 - 2　研究目的举例 2

Aims：To investigate the relationship between depression and self-care behaviors in older individuals with multimorbidity.

还有些作者采用以下格式:The aim of this study was to...。

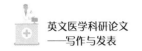
如示例 2 - 3 所示。如果字数允许，有些作者还选择在 Objective 中，给出一定的背景"Background"，如示例 2 - 4 所示。

示例 2 - 3　研究目的举例 3

Objectives：The aim of this study was to assess if menaquinone supplementation, compared to placebo, decreases vascular calcification in people with type 2 diabetes and known CVD.

示例 2 - 4　研究目的举例 4

Study objectives：Major depressive disorder（MDD）is the leading cause of disability worldwide. Its high recurrence rate calls for prevention of first-onset MDD. Although meta-analysis suggested insomnia as the strongest modifiable risk factor, previous studies insufficiently addressed that insomnia might also occur as a residual symptom of unassessed prior depression, or as a comorbid complaint secondary to other depression risks.

此外，还有作者通过说明"研究做了什么"这种形式，给出研究目的，如示例 2 - 5 所示：This study evaluated....。

示例 2 - 5　研究目的举例 5

Objective：This study evaluated the efficacy of smartphone-based, patient-centered diabetes care system（mDiabetes）for type 2 diabetes that contains comprehensive modules for glucose monitoring, diet, physical activity, and a clinical decision support system.

② **研究方法**。这一部分，需要体现研究设计、研究对象、干预措施（如果有）、主要研究变量、测量工具（如果字数允许）、主要统计分析方法，如示例 2 - 6 和示例 2 - 7 所示。有的期刊要求（例如，*J Adv Nurs*），在"方法"之前，单独给出"Design"，如示例 2 - 6 所示）。

示例 2 - 6　研究方法举例 1

Design：Cross-sectional study. Data were collected between April 2017 to June 2019.

Methods：Patients were enrolled from community and outpatient settings and included if they were ≥ 65 years, affected by heart failure, diabetes mellitus or chronic obstructive pulmonary disease and at least another chronic condition. They were excluded if they had dementia and/or cancer. Patient Health Questionnaire-9 was used to measure depression and Self-Care of Chronic Illness Inventory was used to measure self-care maintenance, monitoring, and management. The relationship between depression and self-care was evaluated by performing two sets of univariate analyses, followed by multivariate and step-down analyses. The second set was performed to control for the number of chronic conditions, age, and cognitive function.

示例 2 - 7　研究方法举例 2

Methods：In total, 768 participants from the Netherlands Study of Depression and Anxiety who were free from current and lifetime MDD were followed-up for four repeated assessments, spanning 6years in total. We performed separate Cox proportional hazard analyses to evaluate whether baseline insomnia severity, short-sleep duration, and individual insomnia complaints prospectively predicted first-onset MDD during follow-up. The novel method of network outcome analysis (NOA) allowed us to sort out whether there is any direct predictive value of individual insomnia complaints among several other complaints that are associated with insomnia.

③ **研究结果**。这一部分,需要展示主要研究结果,例如组间差异、相关性分析结果、回归分析结果,如示例 2 - 8 和示例 2 - 9 所示。【注:根据期刊不同,有的要求提供 95% 可信区间;有的不允许提供具体统计值和 P 值】。

示例 2 - 8 研究结果举例 1

Results: The sample (N=366) was mostly female (54.2%), with a mean age of 76.4 years. Most participants (65.6%) had mild to very severe depressive symptoms. Preliminary analysis indicated a significant negative association between depression and self-care maintenance and monitoring and a significant negative association between depression and multivariate self-care. Step-down analysis showed that self-care maintenance was the only dimension negatively associated with depression, even after controlling for the number of chronic conditions, age, and cognitive function.

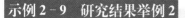

示例 2 - 9　研究结果举例 2

Results：Over 6-year follow-up，141（18.4%）were diagnosed with first-onset MDD. Insomnia severity but not sleep duration predicted first-onset MDD（HR = 1.11，95% CI：1.07 - 1.15），and this was driven solely by the insomnia complaint difficulty initiating sleep（DIS）（HR = 1.10，95% CI：1.04 - 1.16）. NOA likewise identified DIS only to directly predict first-onset MDD，independent of four other associated depression complaints.

④ **研究结论**。这一部分，根据结果给出相应的结论和（或）建议（针对将来的临床实践及研究），如示例 2 - 10 所示。值得注意的是：有些期刊要求撰写完研究结论之后，给出 Impact，如示例 2 - 11 所示。在撰写 Impact 时，需要着重说明：本研究所解决的问题，主要研究发现，以及此研究发现会对什么人、什么地方产生影响。

示例 2 - 10　研究结论举例 1

Conclusion：In multimorbid populations，depression is more likely to be associated with self-care maintenance than the other self-care dimensions. Therefore，self-care maintenance behaviours（e. g.，physical activity and medication adherence）should be prioritized in assessment and focused on when developing interventions targeting depressed older adults with multimorbidity.

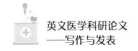

示例 2 – 11 研究结论举例 2

Conclusion： The association between nurses' burnout and perceptions of higher rates of adverse events and reduced safety in clinical practice is an important finding. However，it is unclear whether this was influenced by a negative state of mind，and whether reduced safety and increased adverse events negatively influenced nurses' well-being，thus leading to burnout. Regardless，the association between nurses' burnout and these quality concepts needs further exploration to examine the effect，if any，on burnout and safety，and identify supportive mechanisms for nurses.

Impact： The association between reported burnout and perception of safety and risk of adverse events in Italian pediatric nurses has been reported for the first time. Nurses reporting burnout are at greater risk of intensely negative perceptions of clinical safety and adverse events. This is an important finding as perceptions can influence practice and behaviors. Quality measures in children's clinical environments need to go beyond obvious indicators to examine nurses' well-being as this also influences quality and safety.

2）非结构式摘要。

有些期刊要求提交非结构式摘要，如示例 2 – 12 和示例 2 – 13 所示。虽然此类摘要对书写结构没有特定要求，但它需要包含研究涉及的最基本内容，例如：研究背景、目的、使用到的主要方法、研究结果及结论。

示例 2 - 12　非结构式摘要举例 1

Abstract

Previous studies，which included predominantly Caucasian populations，examined psychiatric and physical illness and associated suicide risk. 【注：以上是研究背景】We used a nationwide database to reassess the findings in an Asian population，and also analyzed the influence of different onset timing of psychiatric and physical illness and the suicide risk. We included 55，630 suicide cases aged 20 - 110 years. Using an incidence density sampling approach，we selected 222，520 controls matched by age，sex，and residence area from 2000 to 2012. We included most major psychiatric and physical illnesses defined by ICD - 9 - CM codes with anatomical classifications. 【注：以上是研究方法】By using conditional logistic regression models with adjustment of covariates，such as patients' marital status and education levels，we found that patients with psychiatric illness had higher suicide risk （adjusted IRR，7. 72；95％ CI：7. 35 - 8. 09）compared with those with neither physical nor psychiatric illness and the risk increased substantially in patients with both psychiatric and physical illnesses （adjusted IRR，18. 35；95％ CI：16. 40 - 20. 86）. Specifically，we found the suicide risk was relatively higher（adjusted IRR，1. 28；95％ CI：1. 10 - 1. 40）when psychiatric disorders occurred before physical illness compared with the other way around. 【注：以上是研究结果】The findings warrant attention to high suicide risk and preventive treatments in patients with both psychiatric and physical illnesses. 【注：以上是研究结论】

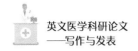
示例 2 - 13　非结构式摘要举例 2

Abstract

Novel biomarkers of type 2 diabetes (T2D) and response to preventative treatment in individuals with similar clinical risk may highlight metabolic pathways that are important in disease development. 【注：以上是研究背景】We profiled 331 metabolites in 2,015 baseline plasma samples from the Diabetes Prevention Program (DPP). Cox models were used to determine associations between metabolites and incident T2D, as well as whether associations differed by treatment group (i. e. , lifestyle [ILS], metformin [MET], or placebo [PLA]), over an average of 3. 2 years of follow-up. 【注：以上是研究方法】We found 69 metabolites associated with incident T2D regardless of treatment randomization. In particular, cytosine was novel and associated with the lowest risk. In an exploratory analysis, 35 baseline metabolite associations with incident T2D differed across the treatment groups. Stratification by baseline levels of several of these metabolites, including specific phospholipids and AMP, modified the effect that ILS or MET had on diabetes development. 【注：以上是研究结果】Our findings highlight novel markers of diabetes risk and preventative treatment effect in individuals who are clinically at high risk and motivate further studies to validate these interactions. 【注：以上是研究结论】

3. 关键词

同摘要类似，提供准确、相关、全面的关键词也很重要。一方面，它有利于编辑根据关键词发现相应的审稿人。另一方面，它可以帮助提高论文的可发现性，多数情况下，检索者会将关键词作为检索词之一。

期刊多会对所提供关键词的数量进行限定，所提供的关键字要能够反映论文的核心内容。一些期刊会为关键字指定 MeSH（医学主题词），这有利于读者在健康领域相关数据库中检索到该论文（例如，PubMed 和 CINAHL）。当然，也可以使用非 MeSH 词，这有利于读者在其他搜索引擎上检索到你的论文（例如，谷歌学术）。对于关键词的选择，有些主编建议：着重 2～3 个关键字，保证在标题，摘要和关键字中重复使用这些关键字，且不要更改术语。

如示例 2 - 14 所示，标题和关键词中均使用到了"psychiatric disorder""suicide"。

示例2 - 14 关键词举例1（关键词与标题使用同样的术语）

Title：Interactions between psychiatric and physical disorders and their effects on the risks of suicide：a nested case-control study

Keywords：suicide；psychiatric disorder；physical illness；bidirectional association；integration care

当然，也有学者建议在标题中尽量避免使用同样的术语，而是使用同一术语的不同表述方式或相关词汇。此外，还可在关键词中给出标题中没有出现的词汇，以对其进行补充；不过，关键词仍需要反映研究的核心内容或特色。多数人在检索时,会将搜索词限定在"标题、摘要或关键词"中。通过以上两种途径,可进一步提高论文的可发现性。

如示例 2 - 15 所示,标题中使用了"difficulty initiating sleep",而摘要中使用了"insomnia",前者是后者的另一个表现形式。类似地,标题中使用了"depression",而摘要中使用了"depressive disorder",这二者均表示同一种疾病/症状。

示例 2 - 15　关键词举例 2(关键词与标题使用同一术语的不同表述方式)

Title：Network outcome analysis identifies difficulty initiating sleep as a primary target for prevention of depression：A 6-year prospective study

Keywords：insomnia; major depressive disorder; prevention; network outcome analysis; multivariate analysis

如示例 2 - 16 所示,标题中并没有给出"mental well-being""personal resources"及"work engagement",但是这些词出现在了关键词中,且反映了干预的特点以及所研究的主要指标。

示例 2 - 16　关键词举例 3(关键词是标题中术语的补充)

Title：Online positive psychology intervention for nursing home staff：A cluster-randomized controlled feasibility trial of effectiveness and acceptability

Keywords：mental well-being; Nursing home; online self-help; personal resources; positive psychology intervention; work engagement

4. 其他重要组成

越来越多的期刊还要求,在给出摘要之后,还有提供"Highlight"或"Statement of Significance"或"Contribution of the Paper",或者在投稿阶段,将这一部分放在一个单独的文档中提交。与摘要类似,应该在撰写完正文之后再撰写此部分内容,简要说明研究的主要发现及对科学研究或临床实践的重要性。提供此内容的主要目的有两个:①让即使没有相关研究背景的读者,也能够明白研究主要发现了什么;②目前,多数人阅读期刊文献,都是通过网络/电子途径,使用此 Highlight 可有利于读者更好地找到你的论文。根据期刊不同,所撰写的内容格式及侧重点有所不同,具体示例如下。

多个护理领域期刊(例如,*Int J Nurs Stud*)要求提交"Contribution of the Paper"。通过两部分说明:①"What is already known about the topic?";②"What this paper adds?"。这两部分,均使用 2～3 个要点进行说明,如示例 2-17 所示。第一部分,着重介绍与你的研究问题相关的进展,**避免对一般研究背景进行概述**。第二部分,介绍你的研究贡献了哪些新的知识、结果、发现,**避免对研究过程进行描述**。例如,以下书写形式就不合适:We examined the effect of an online multi-component positive psychology intervention on well-being and job satisfaction(这是描述过程)。

示例 2-17 Contribution of the paper 举例

What is already known about the topic?

○ Nursing home staff is at risk of stress-related problems.

○ Positive psychology interventions can improve well-being, which is related to various. positive physical and mental health outcomes, and positive organizational outcomes.

○ Acceptability and effectiveness of positive psychology interventions have yet to be tested in nursing home staff.

What this paper adds?

○ An online multi-component positive psychology intervention did not improve well-being, but showed a small effect on job satisfaction.

○ Nursing staff generally show acceptability of a positive psychology intervention.

○ Opportunities lie in creating a positive psychology intervention for nursing staff that is more concise, work-focused, and including some form of autonomy support.

还有些期刊要求给出"Statement of Significance",且有一定的字数限制。比如 *Sleep* 这一期刊,其要求是:①紧跟着摘要给出此部分,总字数不超过 120 字;②对本研究结果的重要性和新颖性进行总结,同时对仍存在的知识空缺(knowledge gap)或未来研究方向进行概述;③语言上要通俗易懂,使得没有此方面研究背景的临床工作人员或科研人员都能够读懂;④避免仅对结论进行重复,避免介绍研究方法,避免引用文献,具体实例,如示例 2 - 18 所示。

示例 2 - 18 **Statement of Significance**

Statement of Significance

The high prevalence and recurrence rate of major depressive disorder (MDD) stress the utmost importance of prevention of first-onset MDD. Using the novel method of network outcome analysis，we identified that，among insomnia complaints，only difficulty initiating sleep（DIS）is an independent and primary predictor of first-onset MDD. Crucially，these findings are of high-clinical relevance，as cognitive behavioral therapy for insomnia is highly effective in improving DIS. Targeting specifically DIS in the treatment of insomnia might aid to combat the global costs of MDD by means of prevention.

还有一些期刊(如 Elsevier 旗下期刊)要求给出"Highlight"。此部分,使用 3～5 个要点(bullet point)对新颖的研究发现和方法进行总结(如示例 2－19 所示)。注意以下事项：①每一条要点不能超过 85 个字符,包括空格；②为了提高论文的可发现性,尽量包含读者搜索时常用的词；③仅原创性论著和文献综述需要提供。

示例 2－19 Highlight

Highlight

○ Frontline COVID－19 medical workers have a high prevalence of sleep disturbances.

○ Females have worse sleep quality than males among frontline medical workers.

○ Further interventions are needed to improve sleep disorders of medical workers.

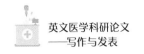

第2节 前言和（或）背景

1. 前言和(或)背景的概述

前言（Introduction）旨在使读者（包括编辑和审稿人）了解本研究开展的大背景（例如国际背景）及开展此研究的原因。对于临床论文，相关大背景可以包括临床实践、研究、教育和政策。就内容而言，前言不可太长，且不应包含太多参考文献。前言中，你可以提到本研究的目的，但是不要直接阐明研究问题，研究问题应该留到下一部分进行介绍。某些期刊可能不需要提供前言，但是为论文提供一个导入性介绍，对于读者一步步进入主题非常重要。养成这样一个好的撰写习惯，对于今后的科研论文撰写生涯具有重要意义。

背景（Background）的撰写围绕着"为什么要开展此研究"开展，对后文起着铺垫作用。背景的内容要以前言为基础，并在此基础上进行扩展。背景中，需要对本研究相关的文献进行回顾、分析和总结，进而说明本领域未知或需要进一步完善（例如，方法学上的不足）的地方，最后顺理成章引出所要开展的研究以及研究如何填补现阶段的未知点或弥补方法学上的不足。

有些人可能会将前言与背景混淆。接下来，将以 *J Adv Nurs* 发表过的一篇论文为例，对二者的联系和区别进行详细说明。

结合本研究的目的：To explore Italian pediatric nurses' reported burnout and its relationship to their perceptions of safety and adverse events，在**前言**中（示例 2 - 20，这里仅截取了代表性语句），作者给出了一段，介绍开展此研究的大背景：WHO 对于职业倦

怠的共识以及职业倦怠在全球背景下的普遍性,最后一句话引出本研究所要关注的重点,为后文的"背景"做铺垫。

示例 2 - 20　前言

Introduction

　　The World Health Organization（WHO）has recently recognized burnout as an 'occupational phenomenon' and, as such, has included it in the 11th Revision of the International Classification of Diseases（ICD - 11）（2019）. They declared burnout a syndrome outcome（Aiken et al. , 2012）... What is clearly known is that burnout is widespread internationally and there are differences in experience, presentation and effects of nurses' burnout across clinical settings... Less is known about whether or not these experiences have an influencing effect on nurses' perceptions of the clinical environment thus accentuating their burnout... The question then is whether or not burnout is a potentiating factor that alters nurses' perceptions of their clinical environmental issues, and affects their performance on the pediatric setting.

　　在**背景**中(示例 2 - 21,这里仅截取了每一段的统领句),作者逐步介绍开展本研究的重要性和必要性。背景的第一段,首先介绍了本研究关注的场所/环境(儿科这一工作场所);第二段进一步聚焦到儿科工作环境下职业倦怠的普遍性;第三段说明职业倦怠可能带来的危害;第四段(最后一段)对既往相关研究进行总结,说明研究空缺(research gap),提出研究问题并引出研究目的。

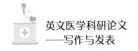

示例 2 - 21　背景

Background

第一段：The pediatric setting is an environment where nurses are thought to be at an increased the risk of burnout.

第二段：However, despite this burnout as a phenomenon appears quite widespread in pediatric settings.

第三段：Several studies have demonstrated relationships between poor staff well-being and poor outcomes including pediatric care (Hall et al., 2016). However, despite this, the emphasis on exploring or improving the safety culture is not necessarily addressed from a well-being perspective.

第四段：Burnout syndrome is a well-documented problem among nurses internationally. Moreover, pediatrics is a high-risk area. Considering the prevalence of burnout among pediatric nurses (de Lima Garcia et al., 2019) and the incidence of errors and adverse events, a question arises as to whether burnout contributes to these in pediatric settings... none to our knowledge involve Italian pediatric nurses. Therefore, the purpose of this study was to evaluate how the presence of burnout among nurses providing pediatric care could influence the perception of the safety of the care.

2. 常见科研术语

撰写研究背景时，需要在总结相关文献的基础上，提出研究问题

(research question),给出明确的研究目的或研究目标(research aim or objective)。另外,有些作者还会明确给出研究假设(research hypothesis)(某些期刊要求必须给出研究假设)。

　　研究问题是开展科学研究的源泉和基础。任何研究都源于一个研究问题,一个研究所开展的所有科研活动(例如,使用的研究设计、研究工具等)都是为了回答这个研究问题。研究问题可以帮助引出后面的研究目的或提出研究假设。此外,前文中所涵盖的前言和背景都是在为引出研究问题做铺垫,而且讨论中也要体现本研究是否回答了你的研究问题。提供明确的研究问题,使得论文在逻辑和流畅性上更加严谨。因此,在撰写研究背景时,给出研究问题是一个很好的写作习惯。

　　与研究问题相呼应的就是**研究目的**。二者既有联系,又有区别:研究目的源于研究问题;研究问题比较宽泛,而研究目的比较具体(研究目的一般要体现本研究想要研究的具体内容)。研究问题可以有几种不同的类型,例如:**描述性、相关性、因果性**。表2-1中给出了研究问题和研究目的的具体例子,进而对二者进行对比。

表2-1　研究问题和研究目的的区别

研究问题(RQ)	研究目的(RA)
How does cognitive function change in patients with diabetes? 【描述性】	To examine the trajectory of cognitive function in patients with diabetes over 10 years.
Do people with better sleep quality have more physical activity? 【相关性】	To investigate the relationship between sleep quality and physical activity in colleague students.
Is cognitive behavior therapy the best way of treating insomnia? 【因果性】	To compare the effect of cognitive behavior therapy with music therapy in the treatment of insomnia in older adults.

此外,在阅读文献时,常常会读到以下词语:Aim、Purpose、Objective,很容易使人混淆。在撰写科研论文时,这几个具有很大的差别。

• **研究目的(Aim/Purpose)**:内容较宽泛,回答以下问题:"What are you doing"或"What do you hope to achieve"(你要做什么?)。研究目的需要反映你开展此研究的原因或意图。

• **研究目标(Objective)**:内容较具体,回答以下问题:"How are you doing it"(你怎么做?)或"The action(s)/steps you will take in order to achieve the aim"(为达到研究目的,你所采取的具体措施或者步骤)。撰写研究目标时,应使用语气较强的动词(collect, construct, classify, develop, examine, measure, produce, revise, select, synthesize),而避免语气较弱的动词(appreciate, consider, enquire, learn, know, understand, appreciate)。此外,还可以借鉴 **SMART 原则**:①Specific(明确):对于你的研究所要完成的内容,要十分清晰、明确;②Measurable(可测量):有利于评估你是否已经达到了研究目标;③Achievable(可实现):一个研究不要试图达到太多目标;④Realistic(切合实际):需考虑实现这些研究目标所需的时间、技能、资金等;⑤Time-constrained(时限性):明确每个目标需要在何时完成。一般情况下,在撰写论文时,仅需要给出研究目的或目标,而不需要同时给出以上所有方面。下面通过示例 2 - 22,对研究目的和研究目标之间的联系和区别进行阐释。

示例 2 - 22　研究目的和研究目标的联系和区别

Aim：The **aim** of this study was to examine the effect of a mHealth application on self-care in patients with diabetes.

Objectives：The **objectives** of this study were to design and validate an eHealth application, test the feasibility of using this application among patients with chronic conditions, and examine its effect on self-care behaviors in 100 patients with diabetes.

并非所有研究都有研究假设,对于量性研究,以陈述的形式表述
两个或多个变量之间的关系,则将其称为**研究假设**。研究假设的提
出基于研究人员对目前相关研究领域知识的熟悉。完整的研究假设
需包括变量、人群以及变量之间的预测关系。研究假设的主要缺点
是:由于先验预测方面的干扰,研究人员可能无法看到预料之外的
结果。

    研究假设与研究问题既有关联,又相互区别。二者都是在研究
开展前需要明确的,其所要达到的目的都是一致的。二者适用的情
形不同:通常,定量研究倾向于使用研究假设(当既往对该主题研究
较少时,多使用研究问题代替研究假设);而定性研究则倾向于以研
究问题的形式表述。另外,研究假设具有方向性和预测性;与研究问
题相比,研究假设更加具体;研究问题提出问题,而研究假设则预测
研究结果。表2-2中,对研究假设与研究问题进行了对比。

表 2-2　研究假设和研究问题比较

项目	研究假设	研究问题
特点	预测某几个变量之间的关系	提出研究所要回答的问题
本质	预测性	探索性
现有研究	有大量研究支持	少量研究
研究设计	量性研究	多用于质性研究、也可用于量性研究
结果	结果范围有限	结果范围较广

    多数情况下,作者并不直接给出研究问题,而是给出其相对应的
研究目的。接下来,将通过几个具体例子,对研究问题、研究目的和
研究假设的撰写进行说明。

    如示例2-23所示,本文中直接给出了研究问题、研究目的和研

究假设。在示例 2 - 24 中,作者直接给出了研究假设和研究目的。另外,有些论文没有直接使用 aim 这个词,而是通过给出研究内容的形式,间接地体现研究目的,如示例 2 - 25 所示。

示例 2 - 23　研究问题、研究目标和研究假设

This study **aimed to** investigate the relationship between burnout，judgement about patient safety and associated risk perception of six adverse events among Italian paediatric nurses.

The **research questions** were：

○ What is the prevalence of burnout among Italian pediatric nurses?

○ Does nurses' burnout impact their perception of the safety of the nursing care that they provide in medical，surgical，and critical care pediatric settings?

We **hypothesized** that a higher level of burnout would be associated with a greater perception of adverse events and a lowered perception of safety in the clinical area.

示例 2 - 24　直接说明研究假设和研究目的

This study's **hypothesis** is that a group of students simulating a bed bath while watching a video will experience improved psychomotor skills when compared to a group simulating a bed bath while instructed by a tutor. Therefore，the **aim** of this study was to test the efficacy of video-assisted bed bath simulation on improving the performance of psychomotor skills of undergraduate nursing students.

示例 2 - 25　间接给出研究目及直接说明研究假设

Here，we **examine** the relationship between patterns of sleep duration over 28 years and measures of cognition，gray matter volume and white matter microstructure in members of the Whitehall II Imaging Sub-Study. We **hypothesize** that consistently meeting sleep guidelines (i. e. sleeping at least 7 hours per night) will be associated with higher cognitive scores，greater gray matter volumes，increased fractional anisotropy (FA) and reduced radial diffusivity (RD) values compared with consistently missing the guidelines，or transitioning in and out of the guidelines over time.

3. 撰写研究背景的技巧

撰写研究背景时,要注意以下几点:

(1) **逻辑性(Logical)**: 好的论文在逻辑上非常严谨,这也会给编辑和审稿人一个很好的第一印象;提高论文逻辑性的一大技巧就是,注意文字的起承转合。上一段落的最后一句话,要为下一段的主题做铺垫。

(2) **简洁性(Succinct)**: 许多期刊对字数都有限制,科研论文(尤其是英文论文)一定要简洁明了,不要有多余的文字。

(3) **相关性(Relevant)**: 部分学者在写作时,为了凑字数,往往会提供许多与本研究无关的内容,这很容易分散编辑和审稿人的注意力,使得他们在读完以后,不知道为何要开展此研究,这也会大大降低论文的可读性和逻辑性。

（4）一致性（Consistent）：同一术语会有不同的表述方式，在撰写的时候要注意使用的一致性。也许你想要 sleep disorder 和 sleep disturbance 表达同一个意思，但对于审稿人来说，它们包含不同的含义；这就会使他们无法理解，进而引起混淆。

（5）明确性（Be specific）：部分学者在撰写论文时，仍保持着比较含蓄的状态。也许你想要表述某个领域没有被研究过，是一个 knowledge gap，但并没有明确说明，默认为读者能够理解。但事实上，读者并不理解你想要传达的意思（尤其是欧美人）。因此，写作时需要直截了当地说明：There is a knowledge gap 或 it remains unknown。使用这样的表述，审稿人就无须猜测，可大大地减轻负担。

（6）清晰性（Be clear）：科研论文的内容需要准确、严谨，因此，所撰写内容不可模棱两可。对于某个论据，要对其进行解释和说明，给出足够的引文支持。

在撰写研究背景时，需要说明开展此研究的重要性和必要性。总结下来，撰写背景的一般逻辑是：

第一段：说明所要研究的某健康问题的发生情况及危害，也就是研究人群。（如果期刊要求提供 introduction，可以将这一段放在 introduction 中；如果目标读者对于所涉及的健康问题很清楚，例如某疾病流行病学，也可以不需要这一段）。

第二段：引出所要研究的结局变量或因变量，说明研究此结局的重要性。

第三段：引出要研究的暴露因素或自变量，对目前相关研究进展进行总结和分析。

第四段：总结目前存在的 knowledge gap 或既往研究在方法学上存在的不足，提出研究问题，进而体现需要开展本研究的必要性。

第五段：说明研究目的/目标或假设，进而引出本研究的**意义**（这一段也可以与上一段进行整合）。

撰写论文还有一个非常有用的小技巧：可以把**每一段话的第一句话作为这个段落的统领句**。要能够做到：把每一段的第一句话连起来读一遍，就能够知道这篇论文想要传达的意思。接下来将对既往的一篇论文进行分析，进一步说明如何撰写研究背景（仅截取了每一段的统领句或核心句）。

本研究的目的是：To describe patient self-care and care partner contributions to self-care and to identify determinants of patient self-care and care partner contributions to self-care at the patient and care partner level. 针对此研究目的，在研究背景中（示例 2 - 26）：第一段，介绍了所要研究的人群及此人群健康问题的普遍性；第二段，介绍了本研究的因变量（self-care）；第三段，进一步介绍了 self-care 的重要性；第四段，介绍了与 self-care 相关的因素（包括自变量）以及仍需进一步研究之处，进而引出本研究的必要性（fill this gap in the literature）。最后一段，给出具体研究目的。

示例 2 - 26 研究背景各段落的书写要点

第一段：Multiple chronic conditions（MCC），defined as the co-occurrence of two or more chronic conditions, have increased worldwide, especially in older populations.

第二段：To reduce the impact of chronic conditions and manage symptoms, patients with MCC perform self-care on a daily basis. Self-care, according to the middle-range...

第三段：Research has shown that self-care in chronic illnesses can improve health-related quality of life and reduce mortality, hospital admissions and costs.

第四段：Several factors are known to influence self-care behaviors in individuals with chronic illness... Few studies have considered illness management as a dyadic phenomenon and investigated self-care determinants at a dyadic level. In addition, those that have considered illness management as a dyadic phenomenon have exclusively addressed self-care of individuals with specific chronic diseases. This study aimed to fill this gap in the literature.

最后一段：The aims of this study were to：(i) describe MCC patient self-care and care partner contributions to self-care in dyads, and (ii) identify determinants of patient self-care and care partner contribution to self-care at the dyadic level.

第3节　研究方法

研究方法(Methods)的撰写不难,却非常重要。其他研究人员也许会参考你的研究方法开展类似的研究;还有一些人可能选择你的论文在组会中进行文献分享;你的论文还有可能被纳入系统综述及 Meta-analysis(荟萃分析)。因此,研究方法必须要严谨、清晰、完整,使别人读到你的论文以后,就能够复制出你的研究。虽然不同的期刊在方法的撰写上有各自独特的要求,但这一部分的撰写可以采用"八股文式"写法。多数情况下,这一部分需要给出:研究设计、研究对象、研究步骤、测量工具、统计分析方法。同时,还要提供其他相关重要信息,例如伦理审查、知情同意、是否进行了注册(实验性研究)。特别值得注意的是,如果研究采用了较新颖或不同寻常的方法,则可能需要提供较强的理由或相应的参考文献进行支持。从期刊编辑和审稿人的视角出发,方法学上存在重大的不足(methodological flaw),通常是稿件被拒的一个主要原因。

1. 研究设计

研究设计(Design)需要简单明了,因此比较容易撰写。对于**非实验性研究设计**,最好说明其是相关性(correlational)还是描述性(descriptive)、是横断面(cross-sectional)还是纵向性(longitudinal)、是回顾性(retrospective)还是前瞻性(prospective)研究。如示例 2 - 27 所示,该研究采用了描述性、横断面研究设计(descriptive, cross-sectional design)。示例 2 - 28 中,该研究使用了纵向性研究(随访 6 年,采用了 4 次重复测量)。

示例 2 - 27 研究设计举例 1

Design and participants

For this study, a descriptive, cross-sectional study was applied using a convenience sample. The study was conducted during 2018 in a private hospital complex in southern Portugal.

示例 2 - 28 研究设计举例 2

Participants

We carefully selected participants from the Netherlands Study of Depression and Anxiety (NESDA), a multisite longitudinal study including four repeated assessments (TO - T3), spanning 6 years in total.

对于**实验性研究设计**,需要说明具体的设计方法;例如:(平行)随机对照试验(randomized clinical trial with two parallel groups)、

交叉随机对照试验（randomized cross-over design）、前后对照试验
（pre-post design）。同时，还可说明是多中心还是单中心
（multicenter or single-center），是否采用了盲法等。如示例2-29所
示，该研究属于随机对照试验，并采用了盲法。如示例2-30所示，
该研究采用了多中心的随机对照试验设计。如示例2-31所示，该
研究采用了前后对照的平行随机对照试验设计，且对研究对象进行
了单盲。目前，多数实验性研究都需要在网上注册其实验方案。此
时，在介绍研究设计时，便可以给出注册号。如示例2-32所示。

示例 2-29　研究设计举例 3

Design and setting

A blind, randomized clinical trial was performed in the
Teaching Skills and Simulation Center at a Federal University
in Brazil.

示例 2-30　研究设计举例 4

Research design and methods

The DPP was a multicenter randomized control trial with
a median follow-up of 3.2 years among individuals at high risk
for diabetes.

示例 2-31　研究设计举例 5

Study design

This was a single, participant-blinded, RCT with a pre-
post design, in which 2 parallel groups were compared,
namely the TENS group and the control (sham-TENS) group.

示例2-32 研究设计举例6

Trial Design and Participants

The study was a 16-week randomized clinical trial (Clinical-Trials. gov identifier：NCT02349477).

多数情况下，论文还会介绍研究开展的场所，例如，医院、社区、实验室等。如示例2-27和示例2-29所示，论文中在介绍该研究所采用研究设计的同时，还介绍了研究开展的**场所**。

有些作者可能汇报的是一个secondary analysis（二次分析），在方法学中，可以引用以前发表过的论文。如示例2-33所示，此研究属于二次分析，引用了该团队既往已发表的研究。特别值得注意的是，在撰写方法学时，要留意自己采用的研究设计存在的局限性，以便与后面的讨论相呼应。

示例2-33 研究设计举例7

Design

This was a secondary analysis of an ongoing multicenter longitudinal study aimed at measuring self-care in patients with MCC and their caregivers; the details of this study have been published previously (De Maria, Vellone, et al., 2019a).

在介绍研究设计或研究对象时，多数需要说明研究是否通过伦理审查（ethical approval）以及是否获得研究对象的知情同意。伦理审查的过程和严格程度因国家而异。一般情况下，期刊并不针对伦理审查所必须遵循的程序进行规定，但是要求说明该研究是否经过相关机构的伦理委员会审查（例如，大学或医院），以确保受试者得到保护,尤其是弱势群体(例如,儿童、孕妇、犯人)。不同期刊针对作者所需要提供的伦理审查证明的要求有所不同,有些期刊仅要求作者说明该研究已经获得伦理审查通过,有些期刊则要求作者详细说明获得哪个机构的伦理审查,还有些期刊要求作者提供伦理审查通过的信件或伦理审查编号。如果后期针对该研究存在任何疑问,则可联系该机构以核查作者所提供的信息是否真实。另外,对于涉及人的研究,还需要说明是否以及如何获得受试者的知情同意。对于不需要获取知情同意书的,需要说明原因。

如示例 2 - 34 所示,本研究中给出了伦理审查的机构以及编号,同时说明了研究对象同意参加该研究。如示例 2 - 35 所示,本研究仅提供了伦理审查机构的名称,同时也说明了已获取书面知情同意书(有时候也可获取口头或网络知情同意书 verbal/online)。如示例 2 - 36 和示例 2 - 37,知情同意被伦理审查委员会豁免。该研究采用了回顾性研究设计且仅收集了匿名数据进行分析。

示例 2 - 34 伦理审查机构及知情同意

Ethical considerations

To conduct the study, permission was obtained from the Regional Ligurian Ethics Committee, on 11 April 2017 (P. R. 075REG2017). Participation in the study was voluntary, and each participant consented to take part.

示例 2 - 35 伦理审查机构及书面知情同意

Ethical approval was obtained from the University of Oxford Central University Research Ethics Committee, and the UCL Medical School Committee on the Ethics of Human Research. Informed written consent was obtained from all participants.

示例 2 – 36　知情同意被豁免

Study design and population

We performed a retrospective, single-center cross-sectional analysis of all patients with a positive finding of *Pneumocystis jirovecii* from January 2000 to June 2017. Written informed consent was waived by the ethics committee due to the anonymized retrospective nature of the analysis.

示例 2 – 37　通过伦理审查且知情同意被豁免

Materials and methods

This retrospective study was approved by our institutional research ethics committee as retrospective data analysis for medical imaging-based diagnoses, and the requirement for informed consent was waived.

2. 研究对象

这一部分需要对研究对象（Sample，Participants，Subjects）进行描述，包括：样本来源或研究对象招募场所、样本量、抽样方法、纳入和排除标准。有些期刊明确要求说明样本量计算方法，所以在研究设计阶段，就要对此方面进行仔细考量。

如示例 2 – 38 所示，该研究介绍了样本来源以及样本量计算方法。如示例 2 – 39 所示，该研究介绍了样本量及研究对象的招募方法和场所。

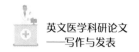

示例 2-38 样本来源及样本量计算

Sample and procedure

The study took place within a large care organization in the Netherlands, counting 17 nursing homes, with about 2000 employees. Taking into account a 25% loss to follow-up, a power analysis indicated that 86 participants divided over two groups were needed to have 80% power for detecting a small-sized effect.

示例 2-39 样本量、招募场所和方法

Participants

We aimed to recruit 404 participants and achieved a final sample size of 410 (205 in each arm). Participants were recruited from the community through multiple channels; for example, the study web-link was sent to contact lists of people who had previously expressed an interest in taking part in sleep research and advertised on websites and social media platforms.

多数情况下,需要对纳入标准和排除标准进行详细描述,以便供其他研究人员参考。有时候,针对某个纳入或排除标准,需要说明设置此标准的原因或相应的支撑文献(例如,**某疾病诊断标准**)。如示例 2-40 所示,研究给出了具体的纳入和排除标准,同时给出了相应的引文进行支持。

示例 2-40 纳入和排除标准(含引文支撑疾病诊断)

Inclusion criteria were (1) aged 25 years and older, (2) meet

DSM-5 criteria for insomnia disorder according to the Sleep Condition Indicator [21], (3) report difficulties with concentration or memory [22], (4) have reliable Internet access, (5) read and understand English, and (6) currently reside in the United Kingdom. Exclusion criteria were (1) screen positive for or report a diagnosis of additional sleep disorder [23], (2) report a diagnosis of mild cognitive impairment, dementia.

另外,对于二次分析,可以通过引用既往发表过的论文,而不再赘述。但是,需要对所提供的信息量进行权衡。一方面,本论文没有必要对既往介绍过的内容逐字逐句进行描述,这反而会增加论文与既往文献的重复率(一旦你的论文发表出来,它就不再属于你而属于出版商);另一方面,论文所提供的内容不可过于简短。对于审稿人来说,论文要为他们提供足够的信息,以便其对论文进行审阅,这一点对于审稿人来说尤其重要。虽然他们可以通过查询你所引用的原始文献获取更加详细的信息,但是很少有审稿人愿意花费更多的时间获取此文献。此种情况下,可以采取以下撰写策略:Detailed inclusion and exclusion criteria have been described in a previous report. In brief...(大致介绍一下纳入和排除标准,而无须给出选择某纳入或排除标准的原因)。如示例 2-41 和示例 2-42 所示,该论文通过引用既往发表过的文献,介绍了研究对象。

示例 2-41 研究对象举例 1

Participants

All participants were members of the prospective occupational cohort study, Whitehall II [13] and the Whitehall II Imaging Sub-Study [14].

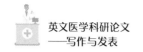
示例 2 - 42　研究对象举例 2

The DPP

The DPP was a multicenter randomized control trial with a median follow-up of 3. 2 years among individuals at high risk for diabetes. Inclusion and exclusion criteria were published previously (14).

3. 研究步骤

研究步骤(Procedures)需要涵盖研究实施过程中每一步所完成的工作。主要包括：研究对象的招募、数据收集、干预实施(如果有的话)。

(1) 研究对象的招募。在符合期刊对于图表数量要求的情况下,建议采用流程图对研究对象的招募进行补充说明。针对**实验性研究**,可以采用 CONSORT 流程图,如图 2 - 1 所示,从研究对象的纳入(enrollment)和筛选(screening)、随机分组(randomization)、随访(follow-up)到最后纳入统计分析(analysis)。在每个阶段,均需要说明研究对象脱落/失访的人数及相应的原因。针对**非实验性研究**,可以采用图 2 - 2 所示的方式,对研究对象的招募过程进行可视化描述。

(2) 数据收集。在介绍此部分时,可从以下几个方面开展：who? when? where? how? what? 说明由谁于什么时间段在哪里如何收集什么数据? 下面将通过实例,进行详细阐述。示例 2 - 43 中,论文介绍了数据收集场所(outpatient and community settings)、时间段(April 2017-December 2018)、人员(Research assistants)。示例 2 - 44 中,论文介绍了数据收集方式(online webpage)、收集内容(questionnaire for...)及具体收集步骤。对于纵向研究,还需要说明

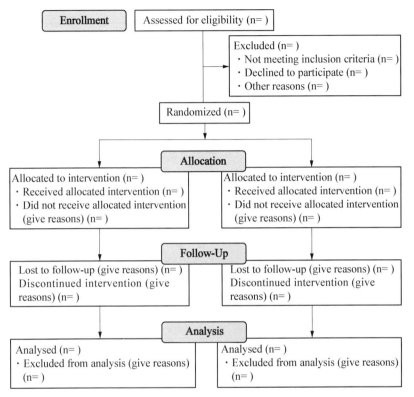

图 2 - 1 实验性研究- CONSORT 流程图

随访时间点。如示例 2 - 45 所示，该研究总计收集了三个时间点的

示例 2 - 43 数据收集举例 1

Data collection

Data were collected from outpatient and community settings in Southern and Central Italy between April 2017 and December 2018. Older MCC patients and their care partners were enrolled by trained research assistants，all of whom were registered nurses.

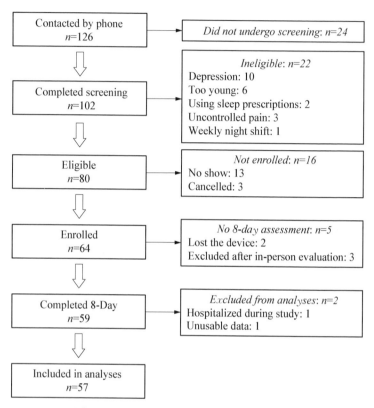

图 2 - 2　非实验性研究-研究对象招募流程图

数据。如果对研究对象进行了补偿,需要说明何时提供的什么形式
的补偿。如示例 2 - 46 所示,该研究在结束时为研究对象提供了 50
美元的补偿。

示例 2 - 44　数据收集举例 2

Data collection

The questionnaire was a version of the one already used

for the RN4CAST study collected in 2017 (Sermeus et al., 2011)... The questionnaire was only available online and data were collected using a secure institutional webpage. Full instructions were given to participants who consented to take part... The online link was accessible for approximately 4 months (September 2017-January 2018).

示例 2－45　数据收集举例 3

Clinical and demographic information was collected by research coordinators. Measures at three time points were assessed：① within seven days before chemotherapy（pre-chemotherapy baseline；assessment 1〔A1〕）；② within 4 weeks of completion of chemotherapy（post-chemotherapy；assessment 2〔A2〕）；and ③ six-months after A2（six month follow-up：assessment 3〔A3〕）. Controls completed study assessments within the same time windows as the patients with breast cancer.

示例 2－46　数据收集举例 4

Participants received 1 h of works payment for completing both（T0 and T1）measurements.

（3）干预方案（Intervention）。对于实验性研究,还需给出具体的干预方案,包括：干预次数、时长、实施者、形式(面对面或远程网络形式)。如示例 2－47 所示,该研究中介绍了实验组的干预形式

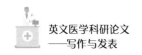

（通过 Sleepio Program 这一线上干预模块）、干预者（animated virtual therapist）、干预次数（six）、干预时长（15～20 min）。另外，这里的干预措施已经在既往的论文中介绍过。所以，作者在引用该文献的同时，又对核心内容进行了概述。对照组未接受任何干预，只是被告知在研究结束以后，可以访问关于此干预项目的网站。

示例 2 - 47　干预措施

Procedures

dCBT was delivered via the Sleepio program，the efficacy of which has been established in several randomized controlled trials（RCTs）[19,25,26]. Detailed information is available elsewhere [19] but in brief，intervention ingredients，covering key cognitive and behavioral strategies，are introduced by an animated virtual therapist in a personalized but automated manner over six 15 - 20 min sessions. Participants also have access to a library of sleep-related articles and an online community forum and can participate in weekly live discussions with a sleep expert. Participants randomized to the WLC arm were informed that they would be provided with access to dCBT at the end of the study（24-week follow-up）.

（4）测量工具（Outcomes and Measurement）。撰写测量工具也有章可循，首先要给出研究变量，然后说明相应的研究工具或测量方法。临床研究相关期刊，尤其是护理期刊，对于测量工具介绍方面要求较高。在介绍一个量表时，要说明该量表包含多少个条目和维度、适用的时间范围、每个条目如何计分、量表如何计算总分、总分是否分级、量表得分的含义。最重要的是，要介绍该量表的信度和效度，尤其是在你的研究人群中的内部一致性信度。如示例 2 - 48 所示，该论文介绍了研究变量（diabetes distress）、量表（DDS）、适用范围（the past month）、包含条目数（17 items）及维度（four domains）、每个条目的评分方法（6-point Likert scale）及量表得分代表的含义（higher score indicates greater level of distress）。最后，介绍了该量表已知的信度及其在本人群中的内部一致性信度（Cronbach's α）。通过这样一个简短却全面的介绍，使得读者对于该研究工具有了十分清晰的认识。当然，对于研究工具介绍的详细程度，因期刊而异。有时候，受字数限制，无法提供太多的细节。如果某测量工具未得到广泛应用或没有相关的引文支持，则需要着重说明为何要选择此工具。

示例 2 - 48　研究工具的介绍

Diabetes distress

The Diabetes Distress Scale (DDS) [25] was used to measure diabetes distress. The DDS consists of 17 items that measure four domains of diabetes-related emotional distress over the past month: Emotional Burden, physician-related distress, regimen-related distress, and diabetes-related intrapersonal distress. Each item is scored on a 6-point Likert scale. A higher score indicates a greater level of distress. The DDS has high internal consistency reliability (Cronbach's α > 0.87) [25]. In this sample, the Cronbach's α of the DDS was 0.94.

以上是对主观问卷的介绍。同理，对于客观测量方法的介绍，也可参照此模板书写。包括所用检验方法、试剂浓度、试剂盒名称及商家。对于常见的测序方法，可以引用既往研究，如示例 2 - 49 所示。

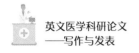

示例 2 - 49　测量方法介绍

Assays and Biomarkers

Urine riboflavin was assayed in the Medical University of South Carolina Clinical Neurobiology Laboratory (directed by R. A.) using standard/calibration curves constructed from known amounts of riboflavin against which unknown amounts of urine riboflavin were calculated by fluorescence detection (448 nm excitation/510 nm emission). Values greater than 1 300 ng/mL indicated adherence. The ‰dCDT was measured with a reference high-performance liquid chromatography assay. 54 Using this international standardized assay, a value greater than 1.7‰ is close to 100‰ specific for sustained heavy drinking in the weeks prior to testing and can be used to corroborate or independently evaluate drinking in clinical trials. 58 Urine ethyl glucuronide (Microgenics Diagnostics) and other blood chemistries, including GGT, were measured with an autoanalyzer.

（5）统计分析方法(Statistical Analysis)。本部分,首先需要详细说明使用的统计分析软件,并给出该软件的版本号、公司和地区。在介绍具体的统计分析方法之前,需要对是否存在缺失值、数据的正态性、是否有离群值等进行介绍。如果有缺失值,说明如何处理缺失值。其次,介绍具体的分析方法,包括统计描述和统计推断。如果所采用的统计方法非常普遍(例如,独立样本 t 检验),则不需进行详细描述。如果采用的统计分析方法比较不常见,需尽量给出引文,说明此方法的出处。最后,需要明确检验水准及检验是双侧还是单侧。对于某些比较复杂的统计分析方法,有些期刊会另外邀请一名统计学专家进行审稿。详见示例 2 - 50、示例 2 - 51 和示例 2 - 52。

示例 2 - 50　统计分析软件及检验水准

All statistical tests were two-tailed, and the levels of statistical significance were set at P<0.05 and P<0.001. We used SAS 9.3 (SAS Institute Inc., Cary, NC) for all analyses.

示例 2 - 51　检查缺失值

A preliminary data analysis was carried out to identify any inconsistencies or missing data. However, given the fixed responses, the only variable with missing data was one of the demographic open-ended items, the work experience, where 13.2% of the answers were missing.

示例 2 - 52　重点介绍复杂的统计分析方法

Modified intention-to-treat analyses were conducted with the Linear Mixed Models (LMM) procedure, including all nursing staff who participated in one of the questionnaires... The LMM analyses included the fixed effects of group (intervention vs. control), and time as repeated measure (T0 vs. T1), and group x time interaction for each well-being outcome measure (i.e., general well-being, job satisfaction, or work engagement).

（6）**其他重要说明。**对于 RCT,在撰写研究方法时,建议参考 Cochrane Risk of Bias 2 Tool 中的条目,这有利于读者对研究质量进行评价。你的论文很可能被其他学者纳入系统综述和 meta-analysis 中，而在系统综述中，其中一个重要步骤就是对纳入文献进行质量评价。

在对 RCT 进行质量评价时，Cochrane Risk of Bias 2 Tool 是目前应用最广泛的工具。该工具主要从以下 5 个方面对某研究的质量进行评价，包括：随机过程中的偏倚［随机分组（allocation randomization），分组隐匿（concealment）］、干预过程中的偏倚（是否对研究对象和实施干预的研究人员采取盲法）、缺失值带来的偏倚（失访情况）、测量过程中的偏倚（测量工具是否合适、测量方式是否合适）、汇报中的偏倚（是否根据预先制定的统计分析方法对数据进行分析）。该量表的具体内容及使用手册将在之后的章节进行详细介绍。

根据以上内容，在撰写 RCT 的研究方法时，需要注意以下几点。

1) 研究对象的分组：说明是否进行了随机分组以及是否采用了分组隐匿（allocation concealment）。当然，这些是在研究设计阶段就应该要考虑到的。如示例 2－53 所示，该论文中明确说明了随机分组方法（按照 1：1 的比例，使用软件进行分组）及隐匿方法（通过协调员 trial coordinator 进行隐匿，科研团队不知道分组情况）。类似地，如示例 2－54 所示，论文中明确说明了随机分组方法（使用软件进行分组）及分组隐匿方法（进行分组的研究人员不是该研究课题组成员）。

示例 2－53　随机分组及隐匿方法举例 1

Randomization and masking

Simple randomization with an allocation ratio of 1：1 was carried out using the randomization function within Qualtrics Survey Software (Qualtrics, Provo, UT) on completion of baseline measures. The research team therefore had no access to future allocations and was unable to influence randomization. Other than the trial coordinator, who emailed participants their allocation, the research team remained blind to allocation. Contact between trial coordinator and participants was limited.

示例 2 - 54　随机分组及隐匿方法举例 2

Students were randomly assigned by a faculty member who did not take part in any of the study's stages using the Random system. This software generated a sequence of two numbers, 1 and 2: group 1 was the Intervention Group and group 2 was the Control Group. The students were assigned to one of the two groups according to the random sequence as determined by the system.

2) 干预的实施: 这一部分,要特别说明是否对研究对象和实施干预的人员采取盲法。**对于药物干预**,多数情况下,可以做到双盲,即:研究对象和干预人员都不知道研究对象接受了哪个干预。如示例 2 - 55 所示,该研究是一个药物试验,采用了双盲,研究对象及研究人员都不知道分组情况(药物组或安慰剂组)。**对于某行为或心理干预**,研究对象不知道自己接受了哪个干预,而干预人员知道研究对象接受了哪个干预。因此,只能做到单盲而无法做到双盲。如示例 2 - 56 所示,该研究是一个行为干预,采用了单盲,研究对象不知道分组情况。干预组接受网络认知行为疗法,而对照组(wait-list control)是在研究结束后,才被授权可以获取网络认知行为疗法相关资源。**对于多数行为或心理干预**,对于研究对象和干预人员,均无法做到盲法。如示例 2 - 57 所示，该研究采用了 open-label（即 unmasked）这一研究设计，论文同时说明了无法对研究对象及研究人员实施盲法的原因。值得一提的是：**针对研究是否采用了盲法，也可以放在"研究设计"那一部分进行介绍。**

示例 2 - 55　药物试验（双盲）

Design，setting，and participants：This double-blind randomized clinical trial conducted between November 2014 and June 2018 evaluated gabapentin vs placebo in community-recruited participants screened and treated in an academic outpatient setting over a 16-week treatment period.

示例 2 - 56　心理行为干预（单盲）

The Defining the Impact of Sleep improvement on Cognitive Outcomes (DISCO) study was an online，two-arm，single-blind，randomized clinical trial of dCBT versus WLC. Participants meeting DSM-5 criteria for insomnia disorder were recruited from the community and screened，consented，assessed，and randomized on a 1：1 basis to intervention or control using the online platform，Qualtrics (www. qualtrics. com). Participants in the intervention arm received access to the dCBT program，Sleepio (www. sleepio. com) [19]，while the WLC group received access to the same program on completion of study follow-up (24 weeks).

Study design and patients：The ISAACC study (Impact of Sleep Apnea syndrome in the evolution of Acute Coronary syndrome. Effect of intervention with CPAP) is a multi-center, open-label, parallel-group, randomized controlled trial of patients with ACS at 15 hospitals across Spain (appendix p 5). Because of the nature of the intervention, the trial intervention could not be masked to either investigators or patients.

3) 数据收集：对于 RCT, 还需要说明数据收集过程中, 是否对数据收集者进行了盲法。如示例 2 - 58 和示例 2 - 59 所示, 数据收集/评估者不知道研究对象的分组情况。当然, 有些研究无法在数据收集过程中实施盲法。此时, 则无须特别强调。

示例 2 - 58   数据收集者进行了盲法举例 1

Data collectors were blinded to participants' group assignment at baseline and follow-up testing.

示例 2 - 59   数据收集者进行了盲法举例 2

A committee, whose members were unaware of the study group assignments, adjudicated the major cardiovascular outcomes specified in the protocol.

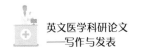

第4节 研究结果

　　研究结果(Results)这一部分,需要简洁明了地给出主要研究发现,确保对所有相关结果进行了汇报,尽可能使用文字与图表相结合的形式报道主要结果,并注意与研究目的相呼应。撰写研究结果时,需要注意:①**避免**针对某结果展开讨论(例如,this finding suggest that...);②**避免**通过文字重复表格中已有的信息,表格与文字应做到相互补充。

　　与撰写前言和背景类似,撰写结果时,也可采用"统领句"的方法,即:第一句话总结此段话(或某表格)想要传达的信息。如示例2-60所示,这一段中的第一句话总结了此段所要展示的内容,并引用了相应的表格(Table 1)。另外,也可采用示例2-61中展示的方式进行描述。

示例2-60　研究结果统领句举例1

　　Clinical characteristics of the metabolite profiling subcohort and complete DPP cohort were similar (Table 1).

示例2-61　研究结果统领句举例2

　　Table 1 shows the baseline characteristics of participants. Mean age was 41.8 years (SD＝12.1, range 16-65 years) and all but one was Dutch.

　　撰写研究结果时,要注意层次性和逻辑性。第一段,多介绍研究对象基本资料;之后的段落,层层递进地回答研究问题或研究假设。如示例 2 - 62 所示,本研究采用了相关性研究设计,研究目的是"To assess the relationship between depression and self-care behaviors in individuals with multiple chronic conditions"。在结果部分,作者逐步向读者展示了与本研究目的相关的结果:5.1 研究对象基本特点。5.2 主要研究结果,包括:5.2.1 自变量与因变量的双变量相关分析(采用了 ANOVA);5.2.2 控制协变量后,自变量与因变量的相关分析(采用了 ANCOVA)。

示例 2 - 62 结果展示方式(相关性研究)

5.1 Participants

5.2 Main results

5.2.1 First set of analyses

ANOVA revealed a significant association between depression and self-care maintenance and monitoring but not with self-care management (Table 4). MANOVA revealed a significant association between...

5.2.2 Second set of analyses

ANCOVA revealed a significant association between depression and self-care maintenance and monitoring after controlling for the number of chronic conditions, cognitive function and age (Table 4).

对于干预性研究,结果展示形式也类似。以发表在 *Diabetes* 上的一项临床试验为例,该研究的目的是:① to identify a unique metabolomic profile associated with progression to type 2 diabetes (T2D) in this population at high risk using a larger sample size—

including validation of our previous findings；② to explore baseline metabolite interactions with the effects of lifestyle changes or metformin。在研究结果这一部分，该论文首先介绍了研究对象的一般资料。紧接着给出了："Baseline Metabolite Levels Predict Incident Diabetes"（与第 1 个研究目的相关），如示例 2 - 63 所示。继而，给出了"Differences in Metabolite Associations With Diabetes Incidence by Treatment Group"（与第 2 个研究目的相关），如示例 2 - 64 所示。最后，给出了"Lifestyle Change and Metformin Effects on Diabetes Incidence in Subgroups Defined by Metabolite Quartiles"（与第 2 个研究目的相关，在上一部分研究结果的基础上进行深入分析），如示例 2 - 65 所示。

示例 2 - 63　研究结果举例 1

Baseline Metabolite Levels Predict Incident Diabetes

IPW-Cox models were used to determine the association between baseline metabolite level and incident T2D with adjustment for age，sex，race/ethnicity，hypertension，FPG.

示例 2 - 64　研究结果举例 2

Differences in Metabolite Associations With Diabetes Incidence by Treatment Group

For assessment of whether baseline metabolite associations with diabetes incidence differed between treatment groups，associations of the 331 known metabolites profiled were assessed using treatment group-specific IPW-Cox.

示例 2 - 65　研究结果举例 3

Lifestyle Change and Metformin Effects on Diabetes Incidence in Subgroups Defined by Metabolite Quartiles

To explore the relationship that baseline levels of metabolites had with treatment effect, we compared the HRs associated with treatment effect stratified across quartiles of metabolite concentrations.

第 5 节　讨　论

科研论文的撰写是一个闭环,完成了讨论(Discussion)的撰写,才算完成了这个闭环。讨论应该将读者拉回到本文的目的,并说明该研究是否回答了背景中提出的研究问题。讨论部分也是将你的研究与既往研究进行对比的一个过程(compare & contrast);通过对比,说明你的研究对某个领域的既有认知有何拓展或对推动临床实践有何贡献。讨论应与本文的其余部分相呼应,尤其是研究结果。**要特别注意: ①避免在讨论部分引入与前文无关的新想法;②避免简单地重复研究结果;③避免对研究背景进行重复介绍。**

讨论的撰写十分具有挑战性,但也有章可循。一般情况下,讨论的撰写可以分为以下几大部分: 概括段;针对主要研究结果进行讨论;说明研究的优势或特色(strengths)及局限性(limitations);研究的启示(对今后科研及临床实践有何指导意义);结论。

1. 概括段

讨论的第一段对本研究进行概括(recap),重新向读者介绍本研究的目的(内容)或说明本研究的新颖性,进而引出主要研究发现,最后说明本研究的意义。如示例 2 - 66 所示,本段第 1 句话,既说明了本研究的新颖性(To our knowledge, this is the first study),又给出了研究的主要目的/内容;第 2 句话对主要研究发现进行了总结;第 3 句话突出本研究对未来临床实践的指导,体现了研究意义。

示例 2 - 66 讨论概括段举例 1

Discussion

To our knowledge, this is the first study describing MCC patient self-care and care partner contributions to self-care and determinants of self-care while controlling for interdependence within the dyads. Our findings confirm the need to adopt a dyadic perspective when assessing self-care and its determinants, since we found that the characteristics of a member of the dyad can influence the self-care behaviors of the other. Routine assessment of such determinants could facilitate the early detection of MCC dyads at risk of engaging in poor self-care.

当然,如果不确定本研究是否是第一个,还可以这么写: To the best of our knowledge, this study was among the first that....。不是所有研究都具有特别突出的创新性;此时,可以采用另外一种概括方式。如示例 2 - 67 所示,本段第 1 句话重新回顾了研究目的;第 2 句话给出了研究假设;进而引出第 3 句话,即研究主要发现。

示例 2 - 67 讨论概括段举例 2

Discussion

The aim of this study was to examine sleep duration trajectories over a 28-year period and their relationship with measures of cognition, gray matter volume, and white matter microstructure. We hypothesized that consistently meeting recommendations for sleep duration (i. e., self-reporting a minimum of 7 hours sleep per night) would be favorably associated with cognition, gray matter volume and white matter microstructure, compared with consistently not meeting the guidelines or transitioning in and out of the guidelines over time. In contrast to our hypotheses, our results did not show any differences in cognitive measures, gray matter volume, or white matter microstructure between different sleep trajectory groups.

2. 讨论的主体段落

讨论的主体段落要与主要研究结果相呼应,避免简单地重复研究背景或结果。需要将自己的结果与既往研究结果进行比较(compare,比较相同点)和对比(contrast,对比不同点):说明你的研究结果在多大程度上支持主流观点;当你的研究结果与既往研究结果不一致时,需要探讨可以解释其差异的原因。通过与既往研究进行比较和对比,说明你的研究对相关领域的贡献,但同时需要避免过度夸大自己的研究贡献。如示例 2 - 68 所示,本研究结果与既往研究结果一致;如示例 2 - 69 所示,本研究结果与既往研究结果不一致。

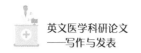

示例 2 - 68　与既往研究结果一致

These results agree with a meta-analysis reporting that the use of simulation associated with technology is effective for health education (Cook et al. , 2011).

示例 2 - 69　与既往研究结果不一致

In addition, previous studies based on the entire Whitehall II cohort found that adverse changes in sleep duration are associated with poorer cognitive function [6]. There are many reasons that our findings may diverge, despite overlapping samples. These include...

　　切忌简单地重复研究结果,要围绕主要研究发现建立一个故事,以说服读者该研究已经达到了相应的研究目的。在撰写讨论时,需要注意:无论研究结果是阴性还是阳性,你的研究都已达到了目的。举个例子,如果你的研究目的是通过 RCT,检验干预组和对照组之间是否有差异。那么,即使研究发现两组没有差异,你也达到了你的研究目的(即,该干预在本人群中未发现显著效果)。当然,如果你的研究假设是:二者会有差异,那么你在讨论中就要着重分析为何你的研究没有发现明显差异。假设你的研究问题是:A 是否比 B 治疗效果要好?如果 A 的效果不佳,则答案为"否",在论文中则需要对此研究结果进行汇报。如果仅汇报阳性结果,则很容易造成发表偏倚。如示例 2 - 70 所示,本研究未发现阳性结果,即研究假设未得到验证。

示例 2 - 70　本研究未发现阳性结果

Such null findings, however, do not necessarily indicate that sleep duration is not important to cognitive health. Rather, our null findings may reflect the limited number of participants reporting extremes in sleep duration within our sample... An alternative explanation for our null results is that it is not sleep duration alone that is associated with cognitive health in aging, but rather a combination of sleep quality and quantity.

3. 研究的特色及局限性

再严谨的研究都会存在一定的局限性,因此,论文需要明确给出本研究的局限性。这不仅可以体现作者对于自己的研究足够熟悉,而且使得论文读起来更加严谨和充实。这些局限性自身也具有价值,它们可以为研究者自己或其他研究人员提供"线索",有利于今后开展更加严谨的研究。此外,越来越多的期刊明确要求:说明自己的研究存在哪些优势或特色(strengths)。例如,研究人群具有代表性、数据收集方法较新颖。任何一个研究的开展都是有意义的,你要向编辑和审稿人推销你的论文,就需要十分明确地提出你的研究有哪些优势或特色及其对科学进步所做出的贡献。

撰写局限性时,要把握好一个度:一方面,不能避而不谈(这会让编辑认为你不够严谨);另一方面,也不能满篇局限性(这会让编辑质疑研究的严谨性和可信度)。一般情况下,在撰写完一个局限性之后,对出现此局限性的原因进行解释(justify),说明在选择此方法时,是经过深思熟虑的。同时,尽量针对此局限性提出改进建议。研究的局限性,一般从研究设计、研究对象(抽样方法、样本量)、测量方法等展开。

如示例 2-71 所示,本研究首先给出了研究的**局限性**,包括①**研**

究设计：研究采用了横断面设计（cross-sectional），限制了研究的因果推断。②**抽样方法**：研究采用了方便抽样法，研究对象来源于社区，代表性不强。同时，作者介绍了为降低此局限性做出的努力：通过从不同地区抽样，减少此局限性带来的影响。③**测量方法**：该研究所测量的概念具有文化差异，研究结果可能不适用于其他国家。④**混杂变量**：研究可能遗漏了重要的影响因素。同时，作者还给出了研究的特色，例如：使用了信效度较高的研究工具、样本量足够大。

示例2-71　研究的特色及局限性举例1

Strengths and limitations

The limitations of the study include the cross-sectional nature of the data, which limits interpretation of causal relationships. Second, participants were recruited mainly from community settings, which may have resulted in a sample with different characteristics from the general MCC population. We tried, however, to counterbalance the convenience sample by recruiting participants from different regions in Southern and Central Italy. Third, self-care and related variables are sensitive to sociocultural influences, so caution is needed when generalizing our findings to other countries. Finally, we considered only a limited number of self-care determinants; research on other possible influencing factors is needed. In particular, self-efficacy and psychological distress should be considered in future studies.

Strengths of the study include the use of theoretically grounded instruments, multicenter enrolment, robust sample size, and the enrolment of dyads similar to those described in different contexts.

在撰写研究的特色和局限性时,要注意二者的顺序。虽然没有硬性规定,但是一般情况下先讲特色,再引出局限性。正如进行评审一样,先总结优点,再提出不足。这种撰写方式层层递进,逻辑性更强。如示例 2 - 72 所示,作者首先介绍了研究的特色,包括:多中心、大样本;且各个中心使用的研究方案一致。以此为基础,提出研究的**局限性**。针对第一个局限性,作者首先对此局限性进行了介绍,紧接着话锋一转,给出了"然而(Nevertheless)",说明这个局限性带来的影响较小。类似地,针对第三个局限性,作者提出了使用"respiratory polygraphy"这种测量方法可能存在"低估 OSA 严重度"的局限性,但是紧接着又解释了采用此方法的原因。

示例 2 - 72 研究的特色及局限性举例 2

The strengths of our study include its multicenter design with a large patient population. All participating centers used the same methodology, and the sleep study was done with the same polygraph model. Nevertheless, this study has several potential limitations. First, we excluded patients with severe ACS and very poor prognosis (cardiogenic shock) as these patients have poor expectations for short-term outcomes. Additionally, we excluded patients with daytime sleepiness who exhibited the most severe OSA. From an ethical perspective, the OSA patient with an Epworth Sleep Scale score > 10 should continue to be treated with CPAP. Our results apply only to non-sleepy OSA patients. Nevertheless, the number of patients excluded for these causes was relatively low. Second, patients in this study were predominantly men; therefore, the results cannot be extrapolated to women. Third, the diagnosis is based on respiratory polygraphy, which could underestimate the severity of OSA. However, full polysomnography monitoring could be a stressful procedure for this high-risk patient group. Moreover, although full polysomnography monitoring is the recommended method for the diagnosis of OSA, data from 2017 suggest that respiratory polygraphy could also be used.

当然,如果研究没有明显的特色,可以不写,直接给出研究的局限性。如示例 2 - 73 所示,作者开门见山,给出了研究的局限性。提出了研究对象依从性不够高(non-completion),但是作者通过引用其他研究,说明自己研究中的依从性不高与既往研究类似,这就缓解了此局限性带来的冲击。另外,作者还针对此局限性提出了改进建议。

示例 2 - 73 研究的局限性

This study had several limitations. Although the noncompletion rate was similar to that for other AUD gabapentin treatment trials[37,38] and a National Institutes of Health National Institute on Alcohol Abuse and Alcoholism-sponsored large multisite study,[47] it should be noted that 13 of 44(30%) of individuals on gabapentin and 18 of 46(39%) on placebo did not complete the trial. Perhaps, adding other supportive counseling or Alcoholics Anonymous attendance could increase retention in treatment. Also, self-reported alcohol withdrawal symptoms prior to study entry might not fully capture the extent of withdrawal severity. In addition, those with complex psychiatric and medical conditions, including history of alcohol withdrawal seizures, were excluded. Furthermore, given its kidney excretion, gabapentin should be studied in patients with AUD with more severe liver disease, a condition in which medications are greatly needed.

4. 研究的启示(Implication)

开展研究的主要目的是推动科学发展、指导临床实践;撰写科研论文还可以为其他研究人员提供研究思路。因此,论文的最后,还需要体现出本研究对未来临床实践或科学研究有何启示和指导意义。通过阅读这一部分内容,读者可以较为清晰地理解如何将你的研究发现应用于临床实践中,也会对未来如何进一步开展此方面的研究有个初步认识。要给出严谨、科学、有针对性的启示,需要对研究目的、研究主要发现及局限性理解得非常透彻。撰写这一部分时,要将其放在这几部分内容的大背景下。下面将通过 2 个例子,进一步说明如何撰写这一部分。

举例 1,本研究的目的:① describe MCC patient self-care and care partner contributions to self-care in dyads, and ② identify determinants of patient self-care and care partner contribution to self-care at the dyadic level. 主要研究结果:① Patients and care partners reported higher levels of self-care monitoring than self-care maintenance and management behaviors. ② Important patient clinical determinants of self-care included cognitive status, number of medications and type of chronic condition. Care partner determinants of self-care contributions included age, gender, education, perceived income, care partner burden, caregiving hours per week and the presence of a secondary care partner. 研究的主要

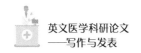

局限性：① cross-sectional nature of the data；② participants were recruited mainly from community settings.

如示例2-74所示,针对以上研究目的、研究结果和局限性,作者给出了以下启示。针对今后的**临床实践**：①同时考虑患者和家属这个二元体(dyad)作为一个整体,对其自我管理水平进行评估,与第一个研究结果相呼应;②对存在高危因素的人提供相应的支持和资源,与第二个研究结果中发现的危险因素相呼应。针对今后的**研究**：①采用纵向性研究设计：与第一个局限性呼应。②进行实验性研究,对危险因素进行干预：与第二个研究结果相呼应。

示例2-74　本研究对未来临床实践和研究的启示

Implications for practice and research

In clinical settings, healthcare professionals should consider the dyad as the 'unit of care', especially in the context of MCC, since self-care for patients and care partners is more challenging due to the possibility of contradictory requirements of the various diseases. Regular assessments of patients and care partners and their self-care behaviours are needed. Support and resources should be offered, especially for dyads with the risk factors we identified (gender, income, education, and availability of a second care partner). Respite care and homecare services should be offered when possible. Additional dyadic studies with longitudinal design are needed in MCC to confirm our results and identify the causal-effect direction. Moreover, intervention studies are needed to modify the risk factors identified.

举例 2，本研究的目的：To assess the relationship between depression and self-care behaviors in individuals with MCC. 主要研究结果：Self-care maintenance was the only dimension negatively associated with depression，even after controlling for covariates. 研究的局限性：①cross-sectional design；②convenience sampling；③secondary analysis；④used a cut-point of five on the depression questionnaire and many of these participants had only mild depressive symptoms.

如示例 2－75 所示，针对以上研究目的、研究结果、局限性，作者给出了以下四个启示。第一个研究启示，针对研究结果和研究局限性 3 给出；第二个研究启示，针对研究局限性 4 给出；第三/第四个研究启示，在综合考虑研究结果及局限性的情况下提出。值得注意的是，有些期刊（尤其是护理学相关期刊）要求使用"Implications for research and clinical practice"或类似的小标题，给出研究启示；有些则不需要这个小标题，而是将研究启示与结论融合在一起书写。

示例 2－75　本研究对未来研究的启示

Implications for research

Future research is recommended to gain a more in-depth understanding of the relationship between self-care and depression in MCC populations. It would be helpful to explore how self-care behaviors change at different levels of depression severity. In addition，future studies should determine if self-care maintenance effectively mediates the relationship between depression and self-care monitoring. With an increased understanding of these dynamics，healthcare providers would be more aware of how best to intervene to improve the outcomes of these fragile populations.

综上所述,研究的特色、局限性及研究启示在撰写上具有一定的连贯性和逻辑性。例如,可以先说明本研究的特色;接着引出本研究的局限性;继而在综合研究特色和局限性的基础上,提出研究对未来临床实践或科研的启示。可以参考以下撰写方式:This study has several strengths... However, there are limitations to this study... Despite the above limitations, findings from this study have important implications for future research and clinical practice.

论文的最后,多是针对该研究给出结论(Conclusion)。有些期刊要求论文单独给出一个小标题(Conclusion),有些期刊则要求将结论放在讨论的最后一段。需要注意的是:结论和摘要不同,结论需要突出主要研究发现及其相关性。如果你在之前的讨论中未单独给出"启示",则在这里需要给出具体的启示或建议内容,这些启示可以针对政策、实践、教育或研究提出。针对你的研究给出相应的结论,切忌引入新的观点。在撰写结论时,始终牢记:很多读者在阅读时,仅仅浏览摘要和结论。因此,要确保结论中所展现的内容具有吸引力。

如示例2-76所示,本论文未给出"结论"这个小标题,而是在讨论的最后一段给出结论。如示例2-77所示,本文中,给出了一个单独的小标题"结论",由于在此之前,文中未单独给出一段展示"启示",所以,在这一部分,作者还提出了本研究对于未来科研和临床实践的启示。

示例2-76　结论举例1

In conclusion, in a large group of patients with ACS and OSA, the use of CPAP therapy had no positive effect on the prevention of recurrent major cardiovascular events. Moreover, the presence of OSA was not associated with an increased prevalence of cardiovascular events.

示例 2 - 77　结论举例 2

Conclusions

The weight of the evidence now suggests that gabapentin might be most efficacious after the initiation of abstinence to sustain it and that it might work best in those with a history of more severe alcohol withdrawal symptoms. To further confirm this, future studies should specifically evaluate symptoms related to protracted alcohol withdrawal during gabapentin treatment. Armed with this knowledge, clinicians may have another alternative when choosing a medication to treat AUD and thereby encourage more patient participation in treatment with enhanced expectation of success.

在撰写结论时,切忌夸大研究结论:你的研究所得出的结论一定要是文中数据能够支持的。对于英语非母语的我们来说,比较具有挑战性,因为不同的单词也许翻译成中文都是一个词语,但其所表达的语气强弱在英文中是不同的。例如,might,may,could,都是"可能"的意思,但是"可能"的程度却是由弱变强。

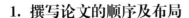

第 6 节　论文的合理布局

1. 撰写论文的顺序及布局

论文的撰写并非一个线性过程。尽管上文的介绍及论文最终的呈现形式具有特定的顺序,但在撰写论文时,可以不按照这个顺序,

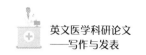

这也是撰写科研论文入门的一个重要技巧。随着撰写经验的积累，每个人都会找到最适合自己的方式。在那之前，本书中介绍的一些规则对于撰写论文经验不足的人员来说，具有指导作用。

撰写论文时，可以先从方法学这一部分开始。研究方法是论文撰写和研究开展前已经确定的，多数不会改变。由于你对这一部分比较熟悉，所以撰写时候就不会觉得不知所措或过于焦虑。一旦开始提笔书写，你就完成了很大一部分工作。完成了方法学的撰写，结果部分就水到渠成。剩余内容的撰写顺序，就按照个人偏好而不同。但是从逻辑上来看，应该先撰写研究背景；接着着手撰写讨论；最后撰写结论和摘要。当然，对于有些作者，可能已经拟定了一个初步的摘要框架。此时，就需要对其进一步完善，以确保摘要确实反映了论文的核心内容。

一篇论文各部分内容所占篇幅也有一定的规则。论文中占据篇幅最大的是背景和讨论，虽然各部分内容所占篇幅并没有硬性规定，但一些编辑针对各部分大约占据的字数给出了建议，如表 2-3 所示。在撰写时，以 500 个单词为单位进行撰写，并以此为基础进行调整。当然，论文的总字数要按照期刊要求，进行相应的调整，尽量做到言简意赅。

表 2-3　论文各部分内容所占篇幅

内容（Content）	字数（Word count）
介绍＋背景（Introduction＋Background）	1 000
方法（Methods）	1 000
结果（Results）	500
讨论＋结论（Discussion＋Conclusion）	1 500

2. 图表相关要求

不同期刊所允许的图表总数量、编号方式及放置位置有所不同。例如,有些期刊要求,图表总数量不超过 5 个。进行此限制的主要原因是:每年的 12 个月内,只允许有限的版面用于出版论文。如果每个作者都使用很多图表,那么这个页面将很快被填满,每期可以发表的论文数量就会降低。如果期刊没有对图表数量进行限定(这种情况较少),就需要根据论文想要传达的主要信息,提供合理数量的图表,以最大限度地帮助读者理解本研究。与文字相比,图表更具视觉冲击力和吸引力。但是,过多的图表反而使论文读起来更复杂。此时,可以将逻辑上和内容上一致的数据展示于同一个表格中。此外,要注意不同的期刊对于图表编号及所放置位置的要求。例如,有些要求图片采用阿拉伯数字进行编号,而有些则要求采用大写字母进行编号;有些期刊要求把表格直接插入文中,有些要求全部放在文末,还有些则要求在投稿阶段单独提交表格。因此,在投稿前,要注意目标期刊对于图表的要求。

各个期刊对于表格的格式和内容也有要求。一般情况下,每个表格都要有一个标题(置于表格上方),标题要清晰简洁、不言自明。在使用表格展示主要内容时,需要确保读者读了此表格,就能够理解你所要传达的信息。所以,要充分、合理运用标注。例如,表格中某个变量(疾病诊断)的各分类加起来大于 100%,这时候就需要在标注中进行说明(某个研究对象有多个诊断)。其他需要在表格下方标注中说明的有:图表中的缩写;表格中不同符号所代表的含义(有些期刊规定,∗ 只能用于表示差异是否有统计学意义);模型中控制的协变量;当表格中所展示的数据是由不同的统计分析方法计算而来时;对于存在缺失值的变量,其样本量是多少。如果在表头中没有给出数据呈现形式,例如:均值(标准差)或频数(百分比),则需要在标注中进行说明。可使用以下方式：Data are presented as mean（SD），unless otherwise specified。另外，尽量在表格中体现出样本量（可以置于标题中或表头中）。如示例 2-78 所示，表格下方使用了标注，对表格中使用到的缩写、模型中包含的协变量、统计学水平等进行说明。如示例 2-79 所示，表格下方使用了标注，说明数据呈现形式 mean（SD）or n（%）、表格中使用到的缩写及统计分析方法。

示例 2-78　表格标注举例 1

* All crude incidence rate ratios (IRRs) listed in this table are shown after matching for sex, age, and area of residence.

** $P<0.001$.

[a]Adjusted IRRs were further adjusted for all of the assessed variables in this table.

[b]Adjusted IRRs were further adjusted for marital status, education, and any psychiatric illness.

[c]Adjusted IRRs were further adjusted for marital status, education, and any physical illness.

[d]Disease codes of the ICD9 are provided in Table S1 (online only).

CI, confidence interval; SD, standard deviation.

示例 2-79　表格标注举例 2

The data are presented as mean（SD）values or n（%）. DBP, diastolic blood pressure; FPG, fasting plasma glucose; SBP, systolic blood pressure. * Two-sample t test. [†] Wilcoxon rank sum test.

　　针对图片,各个期刊对其格式(TIIF,JPG 等)、像素大小、颜色等要求稍有差别。准备图片时,尽量简单;由于多数期刊对于彩色图片会收取版面费,除非必需,一般都使用黑白图片。当然,不是所有论文都需要图片。一些临床医学论文(例如,涉及患者的特殊检查、使用到的干预、3D 打印模型等),会需要图片进行支持和说明。许多护理学论文并不需要图片,需要使用图片较多的情形是:给出研究对象招募流程图或 CONSORT 流程图。每个图片都需要有自己的标题(Figure legend),其撰写要点与表格的标题类似。根据期刊不同,其位置有所不同,但多数要求放在文末。因此,仔细阅读投稿指南十分重要。有些图片的 Figure legend 比较简单,仅需说明图片名称(例如,Figure 1. Study flow diagram)。有些则比较复杂,如示例 2-80 所示。该 Figure legend 中,首先介绍了图片名称;紧接着对图片中 5 个部分(A-E)展示的内容分别进行了说明;最后提供了标注,说明使用到的统计分析方法。

示例 2-80　图片的 Figure legend

Figure 1-Changes in HbA_{1c} levels after intervention. A: After 24 weeks, HbA_{1c} levels were significantly decreased in the mDiabetes group compared with the pLogbook group. B: Per protocol analysis showed a more remarkable difference in the change of HbA1c between the two groups. C and D: There was a more remarkable reduction in HbA_{1c} levels among the patients with baseline HbA_{1c} levels $\geqslant 8.0\%$ ($\geqslant 64$ mmol/mol) and insulin users. E: The reduction in HbA_{1c} was significant among patients in groups C+D but not in groups A+B. The data were analyzed by ANCOVA (A and B) or Wilcoxon rank sum test (C-E). $^{*}P<0.05$, $^{**}P<0.01$, $^{***}P<0.001$.

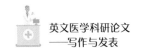
3. 参考文献

参考文献虽然位于文末(看起来微不足道),但却具有重要作用。针对参考文献,有以下几点需要注意。

(1) 确保所引用的参考文献内容新、相关、全面。如果遗漏了最新的研究发现,就可能让审稿人认为你的文献阅读不够全面、你对目前的最新研究进展了解不足。一般情况下,审稿人都是你所在研究领域的专家,有时候审稿人会建议你阅读和引用相关的参考文献,这些文献可能是此审稿人自己既往的研究发现,而你在阅读时没有注意到。有时候,编辑会建议你阅读一些论文,这些论文可能来自你所投的期刊。不管是何种情况,尽量保证在前期准备工作中,对你的研究相关领域的文献进行全面、有深度的阅读和学习。如果发生了以上情况,有两种常见处理方法:如果这些文献与你的论文相关,可以好好阅读并引用这些文献。如果你认为它们与论文无关,则在返修稿件时,针对审稿人的这些建议进行认真答复,说明为什么你认为那些论文与你的研究不相关。切忌直接忽视他们提的这些建议,而不予以回应。如果在某个领域已经取得了一定的成果、发表了一系列论文,那么,在撰写论文时,引用自己的文献很自然,这不仅可以增加你的论文被引的机会,也可以推动/体现自己对该领域的贡献。

(2) 合理地选择所引用文献。有些学者为了引用而引用,而并未深入地阅读和了解其所引用的论文,只是片面地截取了一篇论文中的几句话。这就容易造成论文所展示观点不全甚至是错误。当然,还有些学者仅引用了支持其观点的论文,对不支持其观点的论文避而不谈。这样做不仅不利于开展积极的学术对话、有碍于科学研究的进展,更显得作者对于自己所在领域文献的熟悉度不够。

(3) 引文和参考文献的格式要统一、规范。如果格式不规范,可能在投稿阶段就无法通过初筛,直接就被期刊退回,要求进行修改。

目前,多数人都会使用文献插入软件,例如,Endnote、Zotero。这些软件可针对不同期刊对于文献格式的要求,对文中的引文及文末的参考文献格式进行调整,这可以大大提高工作效率。但仍要注意:即使使用了这些文献插入软件,也要手工对参考文献的格式进行检查和修改。例如:Endnote 所插入的参考文献中,给出的期刊首字母可能没有大写。此外,要注意引文是在标点符号内还是标点符号外(例如:as suggested by a previous report.[1] 或 as suggested by a previous report[1].)。在投稿前,要仔细阅读期刊对于引文格式的要求。有些期刊针对参考文献的格式没有特殊要求,只要一致即可。此时,就可以使用一种你比较熟悉的格式。虽然不常见,但也会有正文中的引文(citation)与后面的参考文献(reference)不一致的情况。撰写过程中,一定要避免此种错误。

4. 论文常用汇报指南

"工欲善其事,必先利其器。"目前,许多期刊要求论文的汇报格式要遵守相关汇报指南。汇报指南是一个结构化的工具,供科研人员在撰写论文时参考,以保证作者在论文中提供了必要的信息。通过这些信息,读者可以清楚地了解到该研究做了什么、发现了什么。这些必要信息可指导今后的科学研究和临床实践,也有利于其他人员将该研究纳入系统文献回顾。针对量性临床研究,有两种常见的汇报指南:CONSORT 指南(https://www. equator-network. org/ reporting-guidelines/consort/)和 STROBE 指南(https://www. equator-network. org/reporting-guidelines/strobe/),前者针对随机对照试验,后者针对非实验性研究。这里将对使用这两个汇报指南时需要着重关注的地方进行简要介绍。

(1) CONSORT。

根据期刊不同,在投稿阶段,有可能会被要求上传 CONSORT

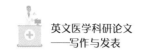
checklist。现已有中文版，详见网站：http://www.consort-statement.org/downloads/translations。在准备此清单时，作者需要提供该指南中每个条目在论文中相对应的页码。根据 CONSORT 指南中涉及的条目，在撰写论文时，应注意以下几点。

1) 论文是对已经做过的研究进行汇报，所提供信息需要透明、真实、准确。 汇报尽量覆盖指南所罗列的条目，但不是每个研究都会严格按照指南中的各个条目来执行。如果研究确实没有遵守某个条目，就需明确说明，而不是让读者去猜。这里最容易忽略的就是：随机（randomization）和盲法（blinding）这两部分，特别是如何进行分组隐匿（allocation concealment）。如果论文缺乏足够的信息，读者就无法对某方面存在的偏倚进行判断。更重要的是，你的论文以后很可能被纳入系统文献回顾，作者就无法判定你的研究存在的偏倚（risk of bias）。如示例 2-81 所示，在本文献综述中，由于原始文献没有提供足够多的信息，该综述无法对该研究在分组隐匿方面存在的偏倚进行评估。关于此方面，本书的**第 5 章**会具体介绍。

示例 2-81　分组隐匿偏倚-不清楚

Allocation concealment

　　Four trials provided insufficient details and were at unclear risk of bias related to allocation concealment.

2) 注意盲法涉及三个方面：研究对象、干预实施者和数据收集者。 多数药物试验可以在以上 3 个方面实施盲法。但是，多数行为、心理或认知等干预，无法实施盲法。此时，在说明无法进行盲法的同时，尽量给出原因。具体写作方法，如本章第 4 节所示。

3) 在多数情况下，实验性研究均需要提前注册。 在进行论文撰写时，需要说明研究是否进行了注册以及注册号。我国的注册平台有"中国临床试验注册中心"http://www.chictr.org.cn/index.
aspx；国际临床试验注册平台有 ClinicalTrials.gov.

**4）该指南中涵盖的许多条目也是在研究开展前需要考虑的（例
如，如何实施盲法，如何进行随机分组）。**所以，在撰写课题或标书
时，也可以参考此汇报指南。

（2）STROBE。

针对非实验性研究（例如，横断面研究、队列研究、病例对照），可
以按照 STROBE 进行汇报，详见相关网站：https://www.strobe-
statement.org/checklists/。与使用 CONSORT 类似，在使用此指南
时，也要保证汇报的真实性、透明性和准确性。在使用此指南时，仅
需针对你的研究所适用的条目进行汇报。例如，如果统计分析中不
涉及亚组分析或交互作用，则 STROBE checklist 中相对应的条目就
不适用（not applicable）。

第3章　原创性论著撰写要点

——基础研究论文

医学基础研究论文是指在医学基础科学研究领域的学术论文，它是将医学基础研究中的新发现和新理论通过精确的语言撰写成的学术论文，是医学科学研究的重要组成。一篇优质的医学基础研究论文，应具有"首发"的原创性，并对研究工作的细节做大量精准的描述，以供其他科研人员参考并在此论文的启发下，完成更有价值的研究工作，共同为人类攻克疾病做出贡献。那么，完成一篇好的医学基础研究论文需要具备哪些要素？本章中，我们将回答以下几个问题。

- 如何撰写简单明了又能传递准确信息的标题和摘要？
- 如何在前言部分有逻辑地介绍研究背景并提出研究问题？
- 如何准确地描述实验方法以供其他科研人员参考？
- 如何清晰地呈现实验结果以帮助读者更好地理解研究发现？
- 如何针对研究发现提供有价值、有深度、有意义的讨论？

第1节　标题和摘要

1. 标题

读者筛选论文的首要依据是标题，好的标题是吸引读者阅读论文的第一步。大部分读者,首先是通过阅读标题来判断一篇论文是否值得继续读下去,读者只有对标题产生了兴趣,才愿意继续浏览摘要、阅读全文。因此,写好标题是医学基础论文撰写的重中之重。好的标题不仅在投稿过程中很重要,而且还会影响论文发表后的引用。

对于此类论文,其标题的书写通常包括三种形式:

(1)叙述型标题。

大部分基础研究论文的标题属于这种形式,此类标题英文结构简单,通常并不会使用复杂从句,多采用一般现在时语态。其主要的特点就是言简意赅地叙述概括整个研究工作的主要发现。这种形式的标题涵盖了研究发现的主要内容,在何种部位、何种细胞中发现了哪些蛋白或基因,标题的叙述能够让读者快速获得论文的重要信息,如示例 3-1、示例 3-2、示例 3-3 所示。

示例 3-1　标题举例 1

SARS-CoV-2 receptor ACE2 is an interferon-stimulated gene in human airway epithelial cells and is detected in specific cell subsets across tissues

---

示例 3-2　标题举例 2

The innate immunity protein IFITM3 modulates γ-secretase in Alzheimer's disease

---

示例 3-3　标题举例 3

Macrophage secretion of miR-106b-5p causes renin-dependent hypertension

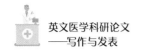

（2）疑问型标题。

此类标题以提出问题的形式来呈现，并可预见研究的主要工作是围绕着回答该问题展开。这种标题的主要特点是更容易吸引读者的注意和兴趣，使读者更有欲望去了解作者所完成的工作。如示例3-4所示，这个标题传达的信息既给出了作者的研究领域，又对传统的公认理论提出疑问，使从事该领域研究的读者更愿意继续读下去，寻找问题的答案。

示例3-4　标题举例4

Does PCNA diffusion on DNA follow a rotation-coupled translation mechanism?

（3）描述型标题。

这类标题通常并未显示出研究的主要发现，其传达的信息主要是介绍给读者新的方法或新的应用，如示例3-5所示。

示例3-5　标题举例5

Impaired hippocampal-cortical interactions during sleep in a mouse model of Alzheimer's disease

虽然标题的书写有多种形式，但好的标题通常能用最简单的形式传达最丰富的信息。标题的书写应具备以下特点：①能够准确地反映研究的主要内容及主要发现，用词得当，不可误导读者且不可过长；②要突出重点，吸引读者的阅读兴趣，使读者阅读标题后对研究内容和发现一目了然；③尽量避免使用缩写，容易给读者造成理解上的困难。其他应该注意的细节，可参考**第2章第1节**。

2. 摘要

摘要是论文的窗口,一篇论文能否吸引读者的关注,摘要起着非常重要的作用。想要写好摘要,首先就要知道什么是摘要。摘要是对论文的内容和要点不加注释和评论的简短陈述,是一个具有独立性和完整性的短文。如第 2 章所述,摘要多放在最后撰写,以保证其准确性。研究目的、研究方法、研究结果和研究结论构成了摘要的四要素。研究目的是要告诉读者为什么要开展此项研究,开展此项研究的目的是什么? 重点是什么? 研究方法是要告诉读者,主要通过什么研究手段和方式来实现这个研究目的。研究方法中,主要是介绍研究对象、研究工作的原理、条件以及完成研究工作所需要的手段等。研究结果中,需要告诉读者,在运用这些研究方法后,研究工作取得了哪些新发现和成果,包括通过调研、实验、观察取得的数据和结果,并剖析其不理想的局限部分。最终,得出研究结论,即通过对这个课题的研究发现所得出的重要结论,包括研究证实的观点、预测其在临床运用中的意义。

不同的期刊对摘要的要求不同,通常情况下,摘要的字数在 250 字左右。字数太少很难说明问题;字数多了又显得冗长。类似地,不同的期刊对摘要的格式要求也不同,包括**结构式摘要和非结构式摘要(如第 2 章第 1 节所述)**。

对于结构式摘要,需要给出研究目的、方法、结果、结论等字眼。研究目的（Aim，Purpose 或 Objective）常采用句式是：To investigate...。研究方法（Materials and methods）需要给出研究所用的动物种类、给药方式及检测手段等,简单清晰地介绍研究工作所采用的方法。研究结果（Results）多采用一般过去时描述,常用高频句式是：Our results revealed that...。结论（Conclusion）多采用一般现在时描述,常用高频句式是：Our results suggest that...。如示

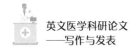

例 3 - 6 所示。

示例 3 - 6 结构式摘要

Aim of study：The aim of this study was to investigate the therapeutic effect of WB on collagen-induced mouse arthritis and explored the underlying mechanism. **Materials and methods**：DBA/1 mice were used to establish a type II collagen-induced arthritis（CIA）model. From the day of arthritis onset, mice were treated daily by gavage with either total glucosides of paeony（TGP, 0. 37 g/kg/d）or WB at a lower（1. 11 g/kg/d, WBL）or higher dose of（3. 33 g/kg/d, WBH）for 8 weeks. The severity of arthritis, levels of cytokines, and the activation of signaling pathways were determined. **Results**：Our results revealed that WB treatment effectively alleviated inflammatory symptoms and prevented bone erosions and joint destruction. It obviously decreased the serum concentration of pro-inflammatory cytokines TNF - α, IL - 6, and IL - 17α, while increased the concentration of anti-inflammatory cytokine IL - 10. Interestingly, the proportion of splenic Treg cells were increased significantly. In vitro experiments showed that WB inhibited the differentiation of osteoclasts. Consistently, the mRNA levels of tartrate-resistant acid phosphatase（TRAP）and cathepsin K（CtsK）, and the activation of NF - κB and JAK - STAT3 signaling pathways in the paws of CIA mice were inhibited by WB treatment. On the other hand, up-regulation of osteogenic genes Runx2, Osterix mRNA, and activation of Wnt/β-catenin signaling pathway along with a decreased receptor activator of nuclear factor κB ligand（RANKL）expression was found in WB treated mice. **Conclusion**：Our results suggest that the therapeutic effect of Wang-bi tablet could be attributed to its inhibitory activity on NF－κB and STAT3 signaling pathway-mediated osteoclast differentiation，and its enhancement on Wnt/β-catenin signaling pathway-mediated osteoblast functions.

许多期刊对论文摘要的结构没有特定要求，并不需要提供诸如 Aim，Methods，Results 和 Conclusion 这样的小标题，但是它仍需要包含研究涉及的这 4 种要素。这种非结构式摘要通常会用 1～2 句话介绍研究背景，然后提出研究目的或者拟解决的问题。这种形式的摘要还会把方法和结果写在一起，介绍通过⋯⋯技术取得⋯⋯发现。如示例 3－7 所示，本文提供了非结构式摘要。

示例 3－7　非结构式摘要

Emerging evidence indicates that osteoclasts direct osteoblastic bone formation. MicroRNAs（miRNAs）have a crucial role in regulating osteoclast and osteoblast function. However，whether miRNAs mediate osteoclast-directed osteoblastic bone formation is mostly unknown. Here，we show that increased osteoclastic miR－214－3p associates with both elevated serum exosomal miR－214－3p and reduced bone formation in elderly women with fractures and in ovariectomized（OVX）mice. Osteoclast-specific miR－214－3p knock-in mice have elevated serum exosomal miR－214－3p and reduced bone formation that is rescued by osteoclast-targeted antagomir-214-3p treatment. We further demonstrate that osteoclast-derived exosomal miR - 214 - 3p is transferred to osteoblasts to inhibit osteoblast activity in vitro and reduce bone formation in vivo. Moreover, osteoclast-targeted miR - 214 - 3p inhibition promotes bone formation in ageing OVX mice. Collectively, our results suggest that osteoclast-derived exosomal miR - 214 - 3p transfers to osteoblasts to inhibit bone formation. Inhibition of miR - 214 - 3p in osteoclasts may be a strategy for treating skeletal disorders involving a reduction in bone formation.

3. 关键词

在撰写医学论文的过程中,需要提供反映论文主题概念的词或词组,用于检索论文,这就是关键词。通常一篇论文的关键词数量不超过 6 个,放在摘要的后面。这些关键词之间用逗号(或分号)隔开,关键词一般是名词(组),个别情况下也有动词(组)。在提交论文之前,可以在 PubMed 中搜索你所筛选的关键词,看看检索到的文献与你的论文是否相关。如果相关性不好,建议优化关键词,如示例 3 - 8 所示。

示例 3 - 8 关键词

microRNA - 193b - 3p, HDAC3, histone acetylation, chondrogenesis, cartilage

第2节　前　言

前言(Introduction)属于论文中比较难写的一部分,好的前言可以让读者迅速把握与论文相关的研究背景以及本研究的目的,从而吸引读者阅读全文,进一步深入了解研究细节。医学基础研究论文中的前言并没有固定的格式和字数限制,但在逻辑和内容上还是有章可循。

前言的第一部分(一般是一个段落)通常会介绍所研究疾病的背景、研究该疾病的迫切性及重要性,并提出以往研究或治疗该疾病存在的不足,引出该疾病研究或治疗的新观点。如示例3-9所示。

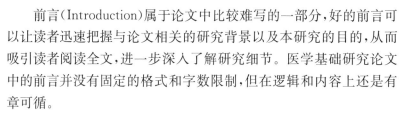

示例3-9　前言第一部分

Osteoarthritis is the most prevalent chronic joint disease affecting knees, hands, hips, and spine; it is one of the leading musculoskeletal causes of impaired mobility (1-3). Currently, no effective disease-modifying drug is available to treat osteoarthritis (4-6) mainly because of the limited understanding of the mechanisms that drive the pathological process at the initiation stage.【介绍所研究的疾病及其危害】Osteoarthritis is characterized by progressive degeneration of articular cartilage (AC), structural alterations of subchondral bone, osteophyte formation, and synovial inflammation (3,7, 8). AC degeneration, the primary concern in osteoarthritis that leads to joint pain and dysfunction, was initially thought to be the only factor driving osteoarthritis development (9-11).【介绍所研究疾病的病理生理】However, treatments targeting only the signaling mechanisms responsible for AC degeneration may be insufficient to halt disease progression (7, 12 - 14). Recent evidence suggests that pathological alterations in subchondral bone also contribute to osteoarthritis development (15 - 23).【提出目前临床治疗该疾病存在的不足，并引出该疾病研究领域的新方向】

前言第二部分(1～2个段落)通常会在上一段提出的新的研究方向或治疗方式的基础上，做进一步扩展。通过引用文献，层层递进地阐述该疾病在最新或者最热点的研究领域所取得的研究进展。紧接着，提出该疾病在上述研究领域还有哪些问题尚未得到解决，进而引出本研究的目的，说明开展本研究的必要性。如示例 3 - 10 所示。

示例 3 - 10　前言第二部分

　　AC and subchondral bone are integrated through the osteochondral junction, which consists of the calcified cartilage zone and subchondral plate underneath. This structure allows AC and subchondral bone to act in concert as one functional unit (8, 18). Bone provides mechanical support for the overlying AC during joint movement and undergoes constant adaptation (modeling and remodeling) in response to changes in the mechanical environment. Changes in the subchondral bone microarchitecture precede AC damage in osteoarthritis in humans (24 - 27). Specifically, in early-stage osteoarthritis, the bone remodeling rate is up to 20-fold faster relative to normal bone, and markers of bone remodeling, such as osteoclast activity, are increased. The rapid subchondral bone turnover observed in osteoarthritis leads to changes in the bone marrow microenvironment and simultaneous neovascularization. Increased subchondral bone angiogenesis, with blood vessel invasion into the avascular cartilage, is an early diagnostic feature of human osteoarthritis (3,28 - 31). This osteochondral angiogenesis not only stimulates early osteophyte development and ossification in the cartilage but also causes innervation of AC, causing joint pain. Consistently, animal studies have shown that aberrant subchondral bone angiogenesis coupled with osteogenesis may contribute to the development of subchondral bone marrow lesions, increased subchondral bone plate thickness, and eventual AC damage (16,32 - 35).【以上内容阐述了该疾病的**最新研究进展**】However, the key factor (s) for the development of pathological subchondral bone angiogenesis and the main source of the factor(s) during osteoarthritis development remain unclear.【提出目前的研究尚未解决的问题】

前言第三部分(一般是一个段落)介绍针对以上提出的未解决的研究问题,本研究完成了哪些研究工作,取得了哪些研究发现,并简要说明本研究的结论和意义。如示例 3 - 11 所示。

示例 3 - 11 前言第三部分

In this study, we tested the role of preosteoclast-derived PDGF-BB in the development of the aberrant subchondral bone angiogenesis during osteoarthritis progression. Using destabilization of the medial meniscus（DMM）osteoarthritis mouse models，we found that mononuclear preosteoclasts in subchondral bone/bone marrow of osteoarthritic joints are stimulated very early in mice after DMM surgery and produce a markedly high amount of PDGF-BB，which activates PDGFR-β signaling to stimulate aberrant development of subchondral bone angiogenesis with coupled osteogenesis as well as nerve ingrowth. We further generated conditional Pdgfb deletion and transgenic mice，in which PDGF-BB is deleted and overexpressed，respectively，in Trap+ preosteoclasts，【以上部分简述了本研究的主要内容，并从体内和体外实验的两个层面介绍了结果】and demonstrated that preosteoclast-derived PDGF-BB is both sufficient to cause and required for aberrant subchondral bone angiogenesis and the resultant joint structural damage and osteoarthritis pain.【简述研究的结论和意义】

综上所示，前言部分虽然没有固定的形式，但却具有很强的逻辑性。在撰写前言部分，可遵循层层递进的规律：介绍疾病背景→提出研究热点→回顾既往文献并介绍发现→提出未解决的问题→简述本研究的主要内容、结果和意义。前言部分字数并无具体要求，但通常情况该部分的字数无须过多，可控制在 500～800 字。

第3节 研究方法

研究方法主要是将研究工作中所使用到的具体实施方案、步骤简明地描述出来。其主要目的是给读者借鉴，为其提供最真实有效的实验信息。通常，论文的读者都是同领域的科研人员，通过阅读论文的研究方法，他们能够完整地重复该实验。

对于研究方法的撰写格式，每个期刊的要求不同。部分期刊要求在研究方法部分将实验过程中所用到的所有试剂全部列出，并注明生产公司。涉及动物实验或人体标本的研究，需要提供伦理方面的证明或知情同意书等。关于研究方法部分在一篇论文中的位置，大部分期刊将该部分放在引言之后，有些将其放在论文最后，有些将其作为论文的"附件"（supplement）。因此，一定要认真阅读期刊的投稿指南，对方法的放置位置进行相应的调整。但无论如何，其宗旨都是让读者能够通过阅读该部分内容，重复出想要做的实验。以下对撰写研究方法时需要注意的细节进行了整理。

① 涉及人和动物的实验，需要提供伦理审查证明和知情同意书，如示例 3 - 12 和示例 3 - 13 所示。

示例 3 - 12　伦理审查及知情同意书

This study adhered to the standards of the Ethics Committee on Human Experimentation at The First Affiliated Hospital at Sun Yat-sen University，China（IRB：2011011）and the Helsinki Declaration（2000）. All participants provided informed consent.

示例 3 - 13　伦理审查证明

All animal procedures，including in vivo animal studies，were approved by the Animal Research Committee of Shanghai Ninth People's Hospital affiliated to Shanghai Jiao Tong University，School of Medicine.

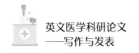

② 对于细胞实验,需要提供细胞来源(并标注公司),如示例 3 - 14 和示例 3 - 15 所示。

示例 3 - 14　方法中说明细胞来源举例 1

Early-passage rBMSCs (passages 2 - 4) were used for the *in vitro* study. The human umbilical vein endothelial cells (HUVECs) used in our present study were purchased from the cell bank of the Chinese Academy of Sciences (Shanghai, China).

示例 3 - 15　方法中说明细胞来源举例 2

Mouse MSCs and macrophages (RAW264. 7cell line) were purchased from American Type Culture Collection (ATCC, USA) and cultured with growth medium consisting of Dulbecco's modified Eagle's medium (DMEM), 10% fetal bovine serum (FBS), penicillin (100 U/mL) and streptomycin (10 μg/mL) in a humidified CO_2 incubator at 37℃.

③ 对于研究中所应用到的试剂,应提供试剂的供应商,并把公司所在的国家及地区一并给出,有的期刊也会要求给出货号,如示例 3 - 16 和示例 3 - 17 所示。

示例 3 - 16　方法中介绍试剂的供应商举例 1

Total RNA from cells, cartilage samples, and cell-seeded scaffolds was extracted using a miRNA Mini Kit (Qiagen, Hilden, Germany) following the manufacturer's instructions

示例3-17　方法中介绍试剂的供应商举例2

For immunofluorescence staining，we incubated the sections with RANK（R&D Systems，Bio-Techne，1：100，AF692），F4/80（Abcam，1：100，ab100790），PGP9.5（1：100，ab10404，Abcam），CD31（Abcam，1：50，polyclonal），endomucin（Santa Cruz，1：50，V.7C7），and PDGF-BB（Abcam，1：50，polyclonal）antibodies followed by fluorescence-linked secondary antibodies（Abcam，ab150120，ab150115，ab150077，ab150078，ab150160）.

④ 对于研究中使用到的常规实验技术,例如 western blot 或 qRT-PCR,可以引用既往文献,但要提供一些关键指标(例如,抗体浓度),如示例 3-18 所示。

示例3-18　实验技术介绍

Western blotting was performed as described previously[17]... Membranes were incubated with primary antibodies specific for HDAC3，SOX9（1：1,000 dilution，Cell Signaling Technology，Boston，MA，USA），COL2A1，AGGRECAN，MMP-13（1：2,000 dilution，Abcam，Cambridge，MA，USA）acetylated histone H3（ac-H3），total histone H3（H3）（1：1,500 dilution，Millipore，Darmstadt，Germany），CD63，CD9（1：1,000 dilution，System Biosciences，Palo Alto，CA，USA），and GAPDH（1：3,000 dilution，Cell Signaling Technology）.

⑤ 对于使用到引物的实验,需要提供基因号及引物的序列。如果使用的引物比较少,引物序列通常会在方法部分直接使用文字描述;如果使用的引物比较多,一般多将引物序列放在表格中列出,如示例 3 - 19 和示例 3 - 20 所示。

示例 3 - 19　文字描述引物序列

The seed sequences were mutated using standard PCR techniques with the following primers: forward 5′ - GAC-ATTATTGGCAGTGGGCCCTGGAAATTCA GCCCTAGC-CCCCCTTGCCCCTTATTT - 3′ and reverse 5′ - AAATAAG-GGGCAAGGGGGGCTAGGGCTGAATTTCCAGGGCCCAC-TGCC AATAATGTC - 3′.

示例 3 - 20　引物序列置于表格中

The relative expression level of mRNA or miRNA was calculated using the 2 - (△△CT) method and normalized to the level of the housekeeping gene GAPDH or U6, respectively. The primer sequences used in this study are listed in Tables S1 and 2.

综上所述,方法部分除了要将研究应用到的技术全部列出,还要将研究方法的一些细节数据给出,例如试剂的浓度、抗体的稀释比例、引物的序列以及细胞的来源等。这些细节数据的完整性决定读者是否能够完整地重复该实验,对于提高论文的借鉴性及可信度至关重要。

第4节　结果和讨论

　　医学基础研究论文的结果和讨论部分是一篇论文的精髓,也是整个研究工作的核心内容。研究结果部分主要介绍整个研究的发现,大部分期刊要求该部分不能引用既往文献,仅单纯地叙述研究结果。研究结果部分虽然没有固定的格式,但通常也具有一定的逻辑性。对于研究结果的描述,多数论文先介绍功能实验的结果,然后叙述机制研究相关结果。对于体内和体外实验的结果,有的作者喜欢一起介绍,有的喜欢分开描述。结果的介绍需要简明,最好能够层层递进,以便读者阅读时能够将前后的数据连贯起来,便于理解。

　　对于讨论撰写,作者需要围绕研究结果进行讨论,但并不是简单地陈述研究结果,而是将研究所取得的发现与既往研究进行比较和探讨。讨论目前所取得研究结果的可能原因,探讨当前的研究结果可能对该研究方向的意义。如果目前取得的研究结果与既往研究结果不一致,需要在讨论部分给出可能造成此差异的原因。对于研究中涉及的一些模型选择及药物应用剂量等问题也可以加以讨论。此外,讨论还需涵盖本研究存在的不足、未来研究中如何避免这些不足以及本研究的意义。大部分期刊要求结果和讨论分开撰写,也有部分杂志要求将结果和讨论整合到一起。需要根据期刊的要求进行相应的调整。现将结果与讨论中的一些撰写要点,进行举例说明。

　　(1) 结果可以分成若干段落,每个段落有一个亚标题去概括该部分结果的主要内容。 亚标题的时态可用一般过去时或一般现在时;段落中的内容多使用一般过去时和被动语态。但是,引出图表中内容时,多使用一般现在时(例如,Figure 1 shows)常用的句式,包括:To further investigate whether...或 We found that...等。如示例3-21和示例3-22所示。

示例 3 - 21　结果举例 1

miR - 193b - 3p regulated the expression of HDAC3 in hMSCs during chondrogenesis【亚标题,使用了过去式】

To further investigate whether miR - 193b - 3p regulates HDAC3 expression during chondrogenesis, we inhibited or overexpressed miR - 193b - 3p in hMSCs. hMSCs were transfected with either miR - 193b - 3p or anti - miR - 193b - 3p and then induced to differentiate into chondrocytes for 21 days (Figure 2).【介绍相应的目的和内容】 The relative expression levels of HDAC3, SOX9, COL2A1, AGGRECAN, and COMP mRNAs were assessed by qRT-PCR (Figure 2A), and HDAC3, SOX9, and COL2A1 protein-expression levels were assessed by western blotting (Figure 2B).【介绍结果,多用被动语态】 The relative expression levels of miR - 193b - 3p on days 7 and 14 are shown in Figure S1.【引出图中展示的内容,多用一般现在时】

示例 3 - 22　结果举例 2

Wnt/β-catenin, AKT and NF-κB pathways are involved in Li-BGC-mediated angiogenesis【亚标题,使用了一般现在时】

To examine the intracellular signaling mechanism responsible for Li-BGC-mediated angiogenesis, HUVECs were stimulated by the 1/32 dilution of BGC and Li-BGC extracts for 30, 60, 90, and 120min, followed by western blotting to detect the activation of Wnt/β-catenin, AKT, and NF-κB pathways.【介绍相应的研究目的和内容】 As shown in Fig. 2A and B，the expression of phosphorylated glycogen synthase kinase-3（p - GSK - 3β），phosphorylated AKT（p - AKT）and NF-κB P65（p - P65）and cytoplasmic β-catenin were significantly enhanced by Li-BGC extracts. 【介绍结果，多用被动语态】

医学基础论文，多会通过与图表相结合的方式，对研究结果进行描述。对于图片，需要格外注意的是 Figure legend 的撰写。Figure legend 是对论文中图片的描述，其主要目的是帮助读者和审稿人快速理解图的含义和结果，不应包括方法细节，通常放在论文的最后。一般情况下，Figure legend 需要包含图片的名称，要求简明准确，要有较好的说明性和专指性；结果中未能表达又必须表达的信息应在 Figure legend 中说明。如图中含有误差线，则应阐述是标准误、标准差、可信区间还是范围。当图片中含有箭头、数字、符号或字母时，则要在相应的位置进行说明，如示例 3 - 23 所示。

示例 3 - 23　图示

Figure 1. Analysis of the relative expression levels of miR-193b and HDAC3 during the chondrogenesis of hMSCs

The relative expression levels of（A）miR - 193b - 3p and （B）HDAC3.（C - E）The relative expression levels of the chondrogenic markers SOX9，COL2A1，AGGRECAN，and COMP.（G - H）The relative expression levels of the hypertrophic markers COL10A1 and RUNX2.（I）The protein-expression levels of HDAC3.（J）Western blots data from three experiments were quantified by densitometric analysis. RNU6B and GAPDH were detected as endogenous controls. The data shown represent the mean ± standard error (SE) of three independent experiments in samples from three different donors. $^*P<0.05$; $^{**}P<0.001$.

（2）**讨论部分并没有固定的格式。**通常情况下，第一段会简要地探讨开展本研究的重要性、必要性、主要研究结果及意义；后面的段落会围绕着研究结果展开探讨，通过与既往的研究结果进行对比分析，体现该论文研究工作的合理性、可靠性及必要性；讨论的最后通常会介绍研究的结论和意义。如示例 3 - 24、示例 3 - 25、示例 3 - 26 和示例 3 - 27 所示。

示例 3 - 24　讨论第一段举例 1

讨论第一段落，再次说明本研究的必要性和重要性。In the process of skeletal development and remodeling, accumulating evidence has demonstrated that cell-cell communication between the vascular endothelium and bone-forming cells is necessary and prerequisite for neovascularization and functional bone formation[3,5]. As the main precursor of osteoblastic cells, BMSCs have been well recognized to play a predominant role in osteogenesis and bone regeneration, and simultaneously serving as a potential regulator of angiogenesis. A broad spectrum of pro-angiogenic factors, growth factors, and cytokines, which have been identified in the MSCs secretome, could influence endothelial cell behavior in vitro and induce angiogenesis in vivo[32,33]. Moreover, a recent study also revealed that the dysfunction of OVX-BMSCs resulted in the decreased secretion of VEGF, along with the reduced potential in promoting the migration, tube formation, and survival of endothelial cells, which has been considered as an important mechanism of impaired angiogenesis in osteoporosis[34]. Hence, the function of BMSCs and BMSCs-ECs communication is of great importance in the initial phase of vascularized bone regeneration. More importantly, a recent study revealed that the chemical signals of biomaterials could boost BMSCs-ECs communication via paracrine secretion and cell contact-mediated mechanisms, consequently resulting in enhanced vascularization and osteogenic differentiation[14]. 【引用以往研究工作的基础上,递进式说明研究工作的重要性】 However, the detailed mechanisms involved in the chemical signals of biomaterials-mediated BMSCs-ECs communication still need to be further elucidated. 【提出研究的必要性】

示例 3-25 讨论第一段举例 2

讨论第一段,简要概述本研究的主要研究结果及意义。 Our results indicate an association between autophagy reduction and apoptosis increase in alveolar process osteocytes of estrogen-deficient rats. Conversely, estrogen replacement increased osteocyte viability by inhibiting apoptosis and maintaining autophagy in these cells,【简述研究结果】 reinforcing the idea that autophagy exerts an important role in the maintenance of osteocyte survival and that the anti-apoptotic effect of estrogen is in part related to autophagy in alveolar process osteocytes. 【体现研究意义】

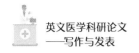
示例3-26　讨论主体段落

　　讨论部分的主体段落,将本研究结果与既往类似研究进行比较。HDAC3 was previously shown to be up-regulated during inflammation and to play a central role in this process[40-41].【列举既往研究结果】In this study, we found that the expression of HDAC3 increased when human PHCs were stimulated with IL-1β, suggesting a biological role that HDAC3 could play in IL-1β-induced PHC responses.【将本研究结果与既往研究进行比较】The cause of increased HDAC3 expression in IL-1β-stimulated PHCs is unclear, but may be attributable to the down-regulation of miR-193b in IL-1β-stimulated PHCs. Previous data showed a positive role for HDAC3 in the transcription of most IL-1-induced human genes. The effect could be mediated by the HDAC3-mediated deacetylation of NF-Kb p65 at lysines 122, 123, 314, and 315[42]. Further studies are needed to clarify the exact function of HDAC3 in IL-1β-induced PHC responses.【列举既往研究,对研究结果进行分析和解释,并引出未来研究方向】

示例3-27　讨论最后一段

　　讨论的最后一段,通常为结论段并说明研究的意义。In summary, the present study demonstrates that Li＋ released from biomaterials exhibits great potential to promote angiogenesis and vascularization. Li-BGC directly promotes the angiogenesis of HUVECs in vitro and new blood vessel formation in vivo. These enhanced effects may be attributed to the activation of Wnt/β-catenin，AKT and NF-κB signaling pathways，while AKT signaling pathway functions as the upstream of Wnt/β-catenin and NF-κB signaling pathways. Moreover，LiBGC further indirectly facilitates the angiogenic capacity of HUVECs by eliciting the expression of exosomal pro-angiogenic factors through the paracrine secretion of BMSCs. Exosomes secreted by Li-BGC-stimulated BMSCs transfer more pro-angiogenic miR-130a to HUVECs，which in turn activate the PTEN/AKT signaling pathway and enhance the proangiogenic capacity of endothelial cells.【总结研究主要结果】Our findings may provide novel insights into the stimulatory role and underlying mechanisms of the chemical signals of biomaterials-mediated communication between BMSCs and ECs in the bone remodeling microenvironment. It is suggested that 3D-printed Li-incorporated bioactive materials may be considered as a promising scaffold for vascularized bone regeneration，especially for large-sized defect repair.【总结研究的意义】

第4章　原创性论著撰写要点

——质性研究论文

　　大家对盲人摸象的故事，一定耳熟能详。有个国王让人牵来一头大象，让几个盲人去摸。过了一会儿，国王问道：你们说说大象长得是什么样子？一个摸到象牙的人说大象长得像萝卜；另一个摸到大象耳朵的人说大象长得像簸箕；摸到大象头的人说大象长得像石头；摸到大象鼻子的人说大象长得像木杵；摸到大象腿的人说大象长得像柱子；摸到大象背部的人说大象长得像张床；摸到大象肚子的人说大象长得像缸；摸到大象尾巴的人说大象长得像绳子。

　　质性研究作为一种研究方法，研究者根据个体对生活体验的描述，分析其中包含的一般性、共性因素，从而揭示现象的本质。如上面的故事中，摸到象牙的人说大象长得像萝卜。这是他的个体体验，是建立在其感官、认识、所处环境和既往经历的基础之上的。通过对"象牙"的大小、质地、温度等的感知，结合自己既往经历中对"萝卜"的体验和认知，他认为与自己过去认识的"萝卜"具有共同特征（如直径约4～5厘米、触感光滑、冰冷等）的"象牙"是另一个"萝卜"。当人们对某一现象知之甚少或现有理论需要修正时，就会选择质性研究的方法。质性研究，或称定性研究、质化研究，是一种在社会学、人种学、教育学、心理学及医学等领域常用的研究方法。由于医学（尤其是护理学）多以"人"为研究对象，关注人的感受和行为，注重人与社会、环境的交互，因此质性研究可以为医学研究提供独特视角，其在健康研究领域中的应用也越来越广泛。

　　本章首先介绍质性研究的概念及特点,其次对健康研究领域中常用的质性研究方法及类型进行简单介绍,最后详细陈述质性研究论文的撰写要点。本章中,我们将回答以下几个问题。

- 什么是质性研究;质性研究的特点及分类有哪些?
- 如何撰写一个"引人入胜"的标题和摘要?
- 质性研究的前言和(或)背景有哪些特殊要求?
- 方法中,应该如何体现研究对象的选择和抽样?
- 质性研究的常用数据收集和分析方法包括哪些?
- 如何撰写一个完整、科学、简练的研究结果?
- 质性研究的讨论如何展开?

第1节　质性研究概述

1. 什么是质性研究

　　如果说量性研究解决"是什么(what)"的问题,那么质性研究解决的就是"为什么(why)"的问题。质性研究(qualitative research)是以研究者本人作为研究工具,在自然情境下,采用多种资料收集方法(例如,访谈、观察、田野笔记),对研究现象进行深入的整体性探究,通过与研究对象互动,对其行为和意义建构获得解释性理解的一种活动。研究者凭借研究对象的主观资料和研究者进入研究对象的处境参与分析资料,找出人类生活过程中不同层次的共同特征和内涵,用文字描写报告结果。

　　质性研究是归纳性的,它通常没有一个先验的概念框架或有待检验的研究假设。质性研究者愿意探索那些被其他研究者相对忽视的领域,或持有怀疑态度地审视他们认为可能不正确或需要修改的领域。因此,质性研究在知识发展中具有产生、指导学科理论的重要作用。护理学中常见的一些理论,如 Ross 的死亡心理分期理论、Swanson 的关怀理论等都是来自质性研究的成果。

2. 质性研究的特点

质性研究是一项严谨、耗时的脑力劳动,其研究设计没有严格的限定,可在研究进展中随研究问题的揭露(uncover)情况来调整。因此,质性研究者需要在研究过程中以积极、开放的心态(open-minded)面对研究问题和研究对象的反应,保持强烈的好奇心和敏感性,随时对研究的内容和方法进行调整。一般来说,质性研究包含以下特点:

- 关注特定的现象或情境,仅对其进行描述,不进行干预。
- 以文字而非数字来回答研究问题。
- 研究方法多样,有时需要对方法背后的哲学思想有一定的了解。
- 质性研究的观点是整体性、归纳性的。
- 多选择目的抽样法(purposive sampling),样本量相对较小。
- 数据收集方法多样且无特定的数据收集工具。
- 资料的收集与分析同步进行,循环往复。
- 数据分析方法不固定,可因研究方法和研究者的不同而有所差异,但都是归纳性的(inductive)。
- 最终形成可以适用于所有研究现象和情境的解释、模式或理论。
- 研究者本人为研究工具,作为"局内人"深入研究情境;因此,质性研究的结果天然地带有一定的主观色彩。

3. 质性研究的类型

质性研究通常是相对量性研究而言,实际上并不是指某一种方法,而是许多不同研究方法的统称;这些方法都不属于量性研究,因而被归为同一类探讨。质性研究包含但不限于现象学、扎根理论、个案研究、民族志、行动研究(action research)、历史研究(historical studies)。以下将介绍护理学中常见的几种质性研究类型。

(1)现象学(phenomenology)。

现象学既是一种哲学,也是一种研究方法;现象学的哲学为方法提供了基础。

1)现象学——一种哲学流派与体系。

现象学,顾名思义,是对"现象"的研究,是关于"现象"的科学。"现象"是"我们所能意识到的东西"或"对我们感官所显现的东西"。它可以是任何东西:一个真实的或想象的物体、一个事件、一个想法、一种感觉或一种情绪。现象学并非简单地了解现象,而是通过对现象的研究,探索现象背后的"本质/要素"(essence)。本质或要素是与某件事的理想或某件事的真实意义相关的元素,也就是给予研究中的现象一般性了解的概念。

正如现象学之父、德国哲学家 Edmund Husserl 所说,现象学"是一门研究本质存在的科学(a science of essential Being)",现象学的目的是建立"本质的知识(knowledge of essences)"。因此,现象学通过对特定现象的观察和探索,分析该现象中的内在成分和外在成分,提炼要素并探讨各要素之间及各要素与周围情境之间的关系。现象学自产生后就以其"回到实事本身"的态度和方法,将众多有着共同见解的哲学家,如 Martin Heidegger、Maurice Merleau-Ponty、Sartre 等联合在一起,形成了 20 世纪最重要的哲学思想运动之一的现象学运动。

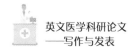
2）现象学——一种质性研究方法。

现象在体验中显示或在经验中被发现。Husserl认为，个体不仅会对他们所参与的世界中产生的各种外部刺激做出反应，他们对于这些刺激含义的认知也会引起个体的反应。现象学着重揭示个体在与他们所解释的世界接触时所构建的意义。因此，现象学研究（phenomenological research）通过相关人员的描述来研究人类的体验（experience），这些体验被称为生活体验（lived experience）。在现象学的意义上，体验不仅包括相对被动的感官知觉经验，还包括想象、思想、情感、欲望、意志和行动。总而言之，体验包括个人生活中所经历或执行的一切。因此，现象学研究的目标是描述或探索个体赋予生活体验的意义（meaning）。现象学研究常被应用于知识相对匮乏的领域，即现有的研究未探明、研究者们不甚了解的领域。

（2）扎根理论（grounded theory）。

扎根理论研究法是由哥伦比亚大学的两位社会学家Anselm Strauss和Barney Glaser共同发展出来的一种质性研究方法。虽然基础理论方法是由Glaser和Strauss这两位社会学家发展起来的，用于研究社会学学科中的问题，但这种方法似乎相当适合医学研究者，比如护理学就非常关注社会交往（或交互）。Field和Morse（1986）提出："建构和概念是以数据为基础的，而假设则是在研究中产生时进行检验的"。他们认为，鉴于护理理论的发展状况，对于护理知识的发展来说，理论生成比理论检验更为关键。

扎根理论是探究人际互相作用中所呈现的社会过程，其研究内容是理论的发现。扎根理论使用理论抽样的方法收集资料，应用持续对比法（constant comparison）分析资料并发展出一种理论，强调研究者要具有理论敏感性。扎根理论法在理论发展中同时使用了归纳和演绎的方法。

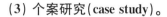

（3）个案研究（case study）。

个案研究最初用于医学教育领域，用来研究患者的案例，后逐渐拓展到心理学、社会学、护理学等领域。个案研究方法是"提供一个或多个案例详细解释和分析的研究"。个案研究讲述的是"一个有界系统的故事"："有界"意味着研究者要识别出系统的轮廓和边界，以此来进行案例的选择；"系统"指的是构成一个有机整体的一系列相互关联的元素，可以是一个人、一个群体，也可以是一个行为、一个事件、一个过程，或一个系统、一个社区、一个家庭或社会生活中的任何单位。研究者应将案例视为包含若干部分并在其环境中活动或运转的整体。个案研究帮助研究者了解到人与人、人与群体，以及人与文化、政治、经济机制的互动关系。

从个案研究的类型上来讲，个案研究主要分为本质性个案研究（intrinsic case study）、工具性个案研究（instrumental case study）以及集合性个案研究（collective case study）。本质性个案研究旨在深度描述一个特定案例，从而理解案例的内在运作；工具性个案旨在通过研究某一个特定对象去了解某一研究问题或疑难，个案只是解决问题的工具；集合性个案同样属于工具性个案，旨在探寻多个个案之间的联系。

（4）民族志（ethnography）。

民族志起源于 20 世纪初的人类学，是一种最传统、最常用的质性研究方法。民族志的字面意思是"关于民族的书写"，其中"ethnos"指"民族、种族和文化体"，"graphia"指"书写或表达"。因此，民族志可被定义为发现和综合描述一个族群的文化，这种研究方法要求研究者通过自身的切身体会获得对当地人文化的理解。民族志研究的本质是决定观察到的行为、事件、情境、仪式等，探讨它们对群体的特殊意义，通过描述和解释文化形式来勾画某个文化群体的肖像（portrait）。

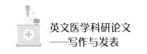

第2节　标题和摘要

1. 标题

标题是一个研究的"点睛"之处,是一个研究吸引读者继续阅读的关键,对于质性研究而言尤其如此。一个引人入胜的质性研究论题,常常需要研究者苦思冥想,从研究中归纳、总结、凝练出最能体现研究成果、最能抓人眼球、最能打动人心的内容加以展现。因此,质性研究的标题常常需要简洁、新颖、有力,使读者在一窥之下即产生往下读的"冲动"。除此之外,质性研究论文标题还需要具有概括性和准确性,这有赖于论文撰写者对研究的熟悉程度、对结果的深入理解和一定的语言功底。

不同于量性研究,质性研究论文的标题常常不那么"完备",不一定涵盖研究的对象、方法和结果三个要素。质性论文的标题中,通常只列出研究问题或重要的研究结果,采用"研究问题+研究方法"或"研究结果+研究问题+研究方法"的模式,前后两部分通常用冒号或破折号连接。标题中展示的"研究问题"可以是一个问句(常以why、how 或 what 开头)或者对研究问题的简要陈述;研究结果可以是一个关键的主题(theme),也可以是一段具有代表性、来自研究对象的陈述或编码(code),常用双引号标出;研究方法可以是一般性的质性研究方法(例如,"a qualitative study")或者更明确、具体的研究方法(例如,"a phenomenological study")。如示例 4-1 至示例 4-5 所示。

示例 4-1　标题举例 1

Compensatory strategies below the behavioural surface in autism: A qualitative study

示例 4-2　标题举例 2

Why rural women do not use primary health centres for pregnancy care：Evidence from a qualitative study in Nigeria

示例 4-3　标题举例 3

Living on the edge：Family caregivers' experiences of caring for post-stroke family members in China：A qualitative study

示例 4-4　标题举例 4

"It's about how we do it，not if we do it". Nurses' experiences with implicit rationing of nursing care in acute care hospitals：A descriptive qualitative study

示例 4-5　标题举例 5

A phenomenological study of the lived experience of nurses in the battle of COVID-19

　　需要注意的是，质性研究标题中，研究方法不一定出现在标题的最后，可以放在标题的前面，有时甚至可以不出现，如示例 4-5、示例 4-6 和示例 4-7 所示。

示例 4-6　标题举例 6

Effective implementation of primary school-based healthy lifestyle programmes：*A qualitative study* of views of school staff

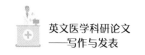

示例 4 - 7   标题举例 7

GP experience and understandings of providing follow-up care in prostate cancer survivors in England

---

由于质性研究的目的是描述一个个体或群体的现象、体验、感受或看法,因此质性研究的标题中常出现一些"特征性"词语或短语,如"体验(experiences)""生活体验(lived experience)""看法、观点、理解(perceptions/perspectives/views/understandings)"" 感 受、态 度(feelings/attitude)"。如上述示例所示,这些词很好地体现了质性研究的研究主题——体验。

2. 摘要

质性研究论文的摘要是研究内容的高度浓缩,体现了研究的精华。在论文其他部分撰写完毕之后,研究者通常会对论文内容(尤其是结果部分)有了整体把握(whole picture),对其中最重要、最吸引人的部分了然于胸。此时,就可以撰写论文的摘要。

摘要的写法并不固定,以文字描述为主,除在方法部分描述样本量、访谈时间外,一般不使用数字。摘要的格式和具体内容需要根据所投稿期刊的要求来决定。质性研究的摘要格式和内容与量性研究的摘要相似(详见**第 2 章第 1 节**):格式可以分为结构式和非结构式摘要;内容均涵盖研究背景(Background)与目的(Objective)、方法(Methods)、结果(Results/Findings)、结论(Conclusions)。摘要可以是一段文字,也可以分段叙述。

下面,将以非结构式摘要为例,对各部分内容的撰写要点进行剖析,如示例 4 - 8 所示。①该摘要首先阐述了所研究问题的现状和目的,强调研究的重要性及必要性。注意,研究目的有时单独列出在小标题下,有时在背景部分的最后点明,通常的写法为"to explore/illustrate/understand/identify the experiences/perceptions/understandings of..."。②其次,介绍了主要研究方法。质性研究摘要的方法多涉及研究的方法学(methodology),即具体应用的质性研究类型、样本抽样方法、数据收集与分析方法等。在示例中,研究者描述的方法内容包括:研究对象("older adults on three levels of health status:healthy and active,managing diseases,or very sick")、样本量("32 participants")、样本来源("from two cities")、数据收集方法("Interviews... audio- and video-recorded")、数据处理("transcribed")及分析方法("Thematic analysis...")。质性研究的方法部分,一般不对观察指标、数据收集工具及统计学方法进行阐述。③紧接着,以高度凝练、概括的语言陈述本研究的重要发现,多展示研究得出的主题(theme)。与量性研究不同的是,质性研究不涉及数字及相应的统计值。④最后,给出了本研究的结论。此部分是对结果的分析、评价和建议。例如,"These results indicate...","Health management programs should..."。

示例4-8 ABSTRACT

Older adult health is often defined in clinical terms. Research has demonstrated that many older adults self-report aging successfully regardless of clinical health status. 【背景】 This qualitative study used claims data to identify older adults on three levels of health status:healthy and active, managing diseases, or very sick, to better understand how health is defined and maintained. 【目的】 In total, 32 participants from two cities were interviewed. Interviews were audio-and video-recorded and then transcribed. 【方法】 Thematic analysis iden-

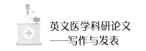

tified five themes: disconnectedness between objective and subjective health; health defined to include psychological and social components; resilience and coping mechanisms indicative of successful aging: social support systems integral to health; and the goal of maintaining functioning. 【结果】These results indicate the importance of individual perceptions of health rather than just counts of chronic diseases. Health management programs should provide holistic approaches to maximize health outcomes and to promote successful aging. 【结论】

还需注意的是,由于特有的哲学基础,虽然也需要客观地反映研究内容,但质性研究天然地带有主观色彩。因此,论文撰写(包括摘要)可以采用第一人称的写法,如"我""我们""笔者"等词汇均可使用。摘要中,尽量避免缩略词和生僻的术语,不用图表,也不引用参考文献。

3. 关键词

与量性研究类似,质性研究的关键词也需要是最能代表研究内容的单词、词组或短语。选取的关键词需规范、简洁、明了,没有歧义。可以在 MeSH 词库中选用,但有时质性研究的关键词无法从 MeSH 词库中选择,只能由研究者自行拟定或参考相关文献拟定。关键词的格式需要根据不同期刊的要求确定,可参考**第 2 章第 1 节**,此处不做赘述。

第 3 节 前 言

前言是论文的开场白,研究所关注的现象和研究问题一般在此部分进行陈述。研究现象是论文将要涉及的领域、范围的总和（包括研究者希望深入了解的人、事、行为、过程和意义）。研究问题是研究现象的具体化，是研究者对研究现象中特别关注和感兴趣的切入点。例如，一项关于失智老人的研究（Defining empowerment for older people living with dementia from multiple perspectives：A qualitative study），研究现象为"失智老人的赋能（empowerment for older people living with dementia）"，这一现象比较广泛，不同研究者可从不同角度探讨，如失智老人赋能的现状及影响因素、赋能的方法、赋能的原因、赋能的意义。在本研究中，研究者将研究问题进一步聚焦于失智老人对赋能概念的认识，即"从失智老人自身、非正式照顾者和医疗卫生专业人员的角度了解赋能对失智老人意味着什么、包括什么（what the concept of empowerment means and includes for people living with dementia from the perspectives of people living with dementia themselves，their informal caregivers，and healthcare professionals）"。

质性研究论文前言（和）背景的写法、内容与量性研究论文类似，通常包括研究的背景、国内外研究现状、研究空缺（research gap）及研究问题产生的思路，具体见本书**第2章**。不同类型的质性研究方法的前言撰写侧重点有所不同，如现象学常侧重于对现象的解释，扎根理论关注理论所要解说的过程或行为，民族志侧重于拥有共同文化的群体，而个案研究则首先介绍个案的独特之处，随后逐渐聚焦于个案的中心特征。

质性研究论文的前言中还常包括各概念的阐述以及为何要选用质性研究方法。例如，发表在 *Geriatr Nurs* 上的一篇论文"A qualitative study to examine older adults' perceptions of health：Keys to aging successfully"旨在"更好地了解各种健康状况的老年人对健康的看法以及这些看法如何影响其健康管理（to better understand how older adults across a spectrum of health describe their perceptions of health，and to consider how their definitions may influence programs to support health maintenance)"。

该论文前言的**第一部分简短地说明了研究背景及意义**。即，健康老化的重要性和应对慢性病状态及适应老化带来的身心变化对于理解"健康老化"和支持老年人群非常重要（"supporting older adults is of great importance"）。这里的写法与量性研究类似。

第二、第三部分对主要概念进行阐述。第二部分对"健康老化"进行阐述：**第一段**说明健康老化的初始定义（"the absence of disease，sound physical and cognitive functioning，and social engagement"），并通过介绍相关理论进一步加深读者对该定义的理解（"The integration of these theories provides a broader definition of health for older adults"）；**第二段**通过介绍健康老化的关键概念之一（自我健康认知"self-perception of health"），引出老年人的主观健康，即健康认知的重要性（perception of health....is a powerful predictor of mortality）；**第三段**提出了研究空缺点：如何将老年人的主、客观健康及老化有机融合（Little is understood about how to integrate the subjective and objective aspects of health and aging into）以及本研究需要采用的研究思路：从整体的观念探讨健康（a holistic view of health）。**第三部分陈述健康的心理社会影响因素**：**第一段**介绍与健康相关的心理和社会因素及其对老年人健康的作用（the psychological and social determinants of health significantly affect the health outcomes and mortality of older adults），**第二至第四段**说明与健康相关的个人因素（resilience，social support 和 independence）以及这些因素对健康及健康认知的影响。

第四部分陈述选择质性研究方法的原因。首先陈述研究目的/研究问题：了解老年人对健康的认识及其对健康支持项目的影响（见上文）。由于研究问题超出了现有的理论模式，且需要从整体、动态的角度来探讨（move beyond the clinical model of health and instead provides a holistic insight into what older adults consider the determinants of health and their health needs over time)，因此，质性研究方法是十分恰当的。此方法能为阐述研究问题提供一个独特思路（This qualitative viewpoint can provide an invaluable perspective of what older adults may need from their own resources，families，communities，or support systems to maintain their health and well-being over time and thus consider themselves as aging successfully）。

当然，有时也可以单独阐述选择质性研究方法的原因，而不与研究目标写在一起。例如，发表在 *Int J Nur Stud* 上的一篇论文——"The impact of moving to a 12 h shift pattern on employee wellbeing：A qualitative study in an acute mental health setting"。在其前言的最后一段，详细陈述了选择质性研究的原因：①研究的问题属于新问题(a new 12 h shift system)；②研究关注的是个体的身心健康(the impact of extended shifts on wellbeing)；③研究问题存在个体与社会环境的互动过程（the demands of a 12 h shift pattern are shaped by features specific to the organizational and workforce context）。

研究目的通常在前言部分的最后，或者研究方法的开端。研究目的的写法与摘要部分的写法类似。有时，亦可提供具体的研究目标。

第4节　研究方法

在质性研究中，研究者作为研究工具，在自然情境下对研究现象进行整体性探究并得出解释性理解。多要求研究对象描述他们的感受、看法、经历或体验，这些感受、看法等主观资料通过多种质性数据收集方法获得，并采用质性数据分析方法进行提取、分析、总结、浓缩

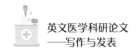

和凝练,最终形成主题或亚主题,展现个体赋予其的意义。

质性研究论文的方法部分通常包括以下几部分:研究方法
(Methods);研究对象(Informants/Participants);资料收集(Data
Collection);资料整理与分析(Data Management and Analysis);伦
理学考虑;可信度。

1. 研究方法

质性研究论文通常在方法部分(Methods)对研究设计进行陈
述,主要陈述所选择的具体方法及选择该方法的原因。这一点与量
性研究论文的方法部分有所不同。

例如,在 *Int J Nurs Stud* 的一篇关于医院急诊科护士对于
"implicit rationing of nursing care"体验的质性研究论文中,研究方
法部分首先介绍了研究设计;随后,作者简单地陈述了选择此方法的
原因。如示例 4 - 9 所示。

示例4 - 9 研究方法

We conducted a qualitative study using *Thorne and
colleagues' approach to interpretive description as a
methodological framework for qualitative health research*
(Hunt, 2009;Thorne, 2008;Thorne et al. , 2004).【研究设
计】Their vision of interpretive description as non-categorical
methodology emerged in response to a call for an alternative
way of generating grounded clinical practice-focused knowledge
that could move qualitative inquiry beyond simple description
to a more abstract genre (Thorne et al. , 2004). The interpretive
description approach acknowledges the researcher's theoretical and
practical knowledge of the phenomenon under study. Moreover,

detailed line-by-line coding is sidestepped in favor of broad questions (Hunt，2009；Thorne，2008；Thorne et al.，2004).【选择此研究设计的原因】

2. 研究对象

根据所要研究的现象和问题，选择具有这一经历或体验并愿意参与研究的个体作为研究对象（Informants/Participants）。样本需要符合一定的"标准"：所选择的参与者需要对某一现象具有特别的经历或体验，以便其分享这些"经验"。此选择并不追求随机，一般采用非概率抽样法，如目的抽样法（purposive sampling）或理论抽样法（theoretical sampling）。抽样过程遵循差异最大化原则（maximum variation），进而有利于直接接触到那些拥有丰富体验的参与者。质性研究的样本量一般较少，通常不超过 25 个（以 15～20 个为宜）；最终样本量的确定遵循**信息饱和原则（saturation）**。示例 4 - 10 对研究对象进行了介绍，包括抽样方法、样本来源、所采用的"标准"。

示例 4 - 10　研究对象介绍

A ***purposive sample*** of 22 participants【抽样方法及样本量】 post MI were recruited from a hospital cardiac rehabilitation unit and from two different communities in Northern Israel【样本来源】. The socio-demographic and cultural characteristics of the participants reflect Israel's population who experienced MI in the past. The participants were chosen from different cultures to obtain a diversity of experiences from different perspectives.【"标准"】

在这一部分,可采用表格或文字的形式描述研究对象的一般资料(也可放在结果部分),以帮助读者了解研究对象及研究适用推广的人群。此时,多采用"一对一"的形式对研究对象进行描述,如表4-1所示。

表4-1 研究对象一般特点逐一列出

N. student	Gender	Age (years)	Year of study	Academic success	Clinical learning experiences	Clinical learning setting	Duration
1	Female	22	1st	Yes	5	Medical department	15
2	Male	21	2nd	Yes	1	Week surgery	15

3. 资料收集

质性研究中最常用的资料收集方法是访谈法,包括深度访谈法(in-depth interview)和焦点小组访谈法(focus group interview);另外,还可通过观察法(observation)、田野笔记(field notes)、日记(diary)等收集特殊经历的书面描述、文学艺术作品、影像资料等。

(1) 深度访谈法(in-depth interview)。

深度访谈法的目的不在于寻求某一问题的特定答案或对某一假设进行验证,而在于了解他人经历、经验的内在意义。研究者引导、鼓励研究对象用自己的语言表达自己对于研究现象的经历、看法和感受;从研究对象的视角出发,获得他们对研究现象深入细致的描述及他们对意义的解释,从而获得一个具有整体性、比较宽广的视野。资料收集一直持续到研究者相信所获取信息已达到饱和状态(saturation),也就是从研究对象那里无法获取新的信息/主题。

（2）焦点团体访谈（focus group interview）。

小组访谈法是指**焦点团体访谈**（focus group interview），是一种最常见的集体访谈方式。1～2 个研究者同时对一群人进行访谈，通过群体成员之间的互动对研究的"焦点"进行探讨。这里的"焦点"是指一个开放性的问题（open-ended question）。此方法不仅涉及研究者与访谈者一对一的有序谈话，还鼓励参与者之间相互交谈。因此，研究者可以将访谈本身作为研究的对象，通过观察参与者之间的互动行为来了解他们在个体访谈中不会表现出来的行为。此方法通过相互讨论、补充和纠正研究焦点，往往比个体访谈更具深度和广度；适用于了解看法或意见而非个性的故事，不适用于一些涉及隐私或敏感的话题。

根据研究者对访谈的"控制程度"，访谈又可分为结构式访谈（structured interview）、半结构式访谈（semi-structured interview）及无结构式访谈（unstructured interview）。质性研究中的访谈指的就是后两种。根据研究设计类型及对研究问题的了解程度，可选择无结构式或半结构式访谈。

无结构式访谈一般以一个开场问题（opening question）作为访谈的开端，根据研究对象的回答来不断地追问。例如，既往研究中，研究者想要了解脑卒中家庭照顾者的照顾意义。此时，研究者对于"家庭照顾（family caregiving）"了解很少，因此选择无结构式访谈，设计开场问题为"What is it like for you to care for your family member who has a stroke？"。

半结构式访谈常常需要提前设计访谈提纲（interview guide），访谈提纲的制定来源于文献资料、专家意见或预访谈。访谈提纲多为开放式问题（open-ended question），且不以简单的"是"或"否"来回答的问题。如示例 4 - 11 所示，资料收集部分，作者首先说明了数据收集方法、访谈提纲制定方法、问题形式；研究者还随时根据研究对象的回答来追问并且设计了"提词（prompts）"来鼓励被访谈者进行分

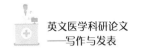

享。在段落的最后，作者给出了示例问题和提词。

示例4-11 资料收集：半结构式访谈

A semi-structured in-depth interview guide was developed based on scientific literature，expert peer review by two cardiologist physicians，two cardiology nurses，and three qualitative researchers.【数据收集方法、访谈提纲制定方法】 The interview guide included a set of 44 predetermined，open-ended questions including prompts，in a way that encouraged participants to convey their viewpoints.【问题形式、提词】In addition，other questions emerged from the dialog.【追问】... Examples of questions：What in your opinion helps people preserve their health? From your experience，what works best for you? (Prompts：what kind of help is most meaningful，who plays a significant role? who else?). What of all the things you want to do for your health is more difficult for you to do? (Prompts：What else? Why? How do you explain it?)【问题示例】

在资料收集部分，还需陈述资料收集的时间、地点、联系人及数据收集者、收集方式、收集后的数据处理及知情同意。如示例4-12所示：访谈场所为"心脏康复单元(cardiac rehabilitation unit)"或"由研究对象选择的场所，如家或咖啡馆(place of convenience to the participants)"；访谈时间为"患者预定的复诊前后(before or after participants' scheduled follow-up visits)或访谈对象方便的时间"；联系人为"心脏康复护士(cardiac rehabilitation nurse)"；并"获取研究对象知情同意(asked their permission to participate)"。**数据收集者**

为"研究第一负责人和 4 个护理学生（The primary investigator conducted ten interviews，and supervised four nursing students，who conducted twelve more interviews）"；采用"录音形式（all interviews recorded）"记录。数据整理包括原始数据处理及转录："主要用阿拉伯语收集原始资料，部分用希伯来语收集（Six interviews were conducted in Arabic... The remaining interviews were conducted in Hebrew）"；对于数据处理，"研究对象的原话最终全部由第一负责人翻译为英文，并由一位双语研究者进行回译（All the participants' quotations were translated into English by the primary investigator，and back translated by one of the bilingual co-researchers to ensure that meaning was retained）"。最后，还提到研究使用到的其他资料收集方法"田野笔记（Field notes）"。

示例 4 - 12　资料收集方法和过程

The hospital interviews took place in the cardiac rehabilitation unit，before or after participants' scheduled follow-up visits. The cardiac rehabilitation nurse contacted the participants by telephone，prior to their scheduled clinic visit，and asked their permission to participate in the study interview. The community interviews were scheduled by phone calls or face to face，at a time and place of convenience to the participants（i. e.，home or coffee shop）. Interviews lasted approximately 45 - 60 min. The primary investigator conducted ten interviews，and supervised four nursing students，who conducted twelve more interviews as partial requirement of a qualitative seminar. Six interviews were conducted in Arabic，then translated into Hebrew by two Arabic-speaking nursing students who were also proficient in

Hebrew; Hebrew is required for advanced nursing students in higher education. The remaining interviews were conducted in Hebrew. All the participants' quotations were translated into English by the primary investigator, and back-translated by one of the bilingual co-researchers to ensure that meaning was retained. All translations were edited by a professional Israeli-American editor. Field notes were collected and all interviews were recorded and transcribed.

此外,在资料收集过程中,需及时对访谈内容进行转录,进而评估是否已达到数据饱和。若数据达到饱和,多停止资料收集。如示例 4 - 13 所示。

示例 4 - 13 资料收集至数据饱和

Records were immediately transcribed verbatim aiming at continuing evaluating the saturation, by sharing the data collected among researchers. When the data saturation was achieved as judged independently by three researchers, the data collection process ended.

4. 资料整理与分析

(1) 资料整理。

资料整理是分析的前提,始于数据收集阶段;数据分析建立在良好的资料整理基础之上。资料整理包括**转录(transcribe)和沉浸(immerse)**。转录,即将访谈录音(包括语言、语气词、音调、沉默、哭笑等）、田野笔记等转为文本的过程。沉浸，即为深入资料中，研究者通过对访谈录音及转录文本反复听及阅读（listening and re-listening，reading and re-reading），与资料"互动"，对资料产生整体把握（a holistic view）和熟悉（be familiar with the data），将自己"沉浸"在资料中（be immersed in the data）。部分研究（描述现象学）还需要研究者在此过程摒弃自己对研究现象既有认识和理解（preunderstanding），通常通过使用括号注解（bracketing）的方法，采用写备忘录（memo）或日记（dairy）的形式来实现。

在这一部分，需要说明参与资料整理和分析的人员以及涉及的具体步骤。如示例4-14所示，作者首先说明数据分析人员：主要研究者（primary investigator）和其他不直接参与访谈的合作者（co-researchers，not directly connected to the interview process）。主要研究者将录音和田野笔记进行整理，转录为22份"文本（transcripts）"，并分析了全部文本；其他研究者分为两组，每组独立分析一半的文本。研究小组就分析结果进行比较、讨论并最终达成一致意见。又如示例4-15所示，该研究中，作者通过反复阅读转录文本对所获资料有所熟悉。

示例4-14 资料整理和分析

All the interview transcripts and the field notes were analyzed by the primary investigator. The co-researchers, not directly connected to the interview process, independently analyzed half of the transcripts. The 22 interview transcripts were randomly divided into two groups (i. e., even and odd) and each group included five interviews with cardiac rehabilitation participants and six with community participants. Findings were compared and discussed by the research team during organized meetings until consensus was reached.

示例 4 - 15　沉浸在资料中

The transcripts were read and re-read to obtain a global
view and to familiarise the reader with the data.

(2) 资料分析。

质性研究的资料分析与资料收集同步进行,当资料收集开始时,
资料分析也随之开展。资料分析结果决定是否需要继续收集资料。
资料分析是质性研究中最具挑战的环节,其目的是既要保存每个访
谈对象个体生活经验的独特性,又能对研究中的现象产生了解。

质性研究的数据分析方法大致可分为两类:一类来源或遵循固
定的理论或认知论立场(theoretical or epistemological position)或在
该理论或认知论框架下的具体方法(manifestations of the method),
例如现象学中的诠释现象学分析(interpretative phenomenological
analysis)、Giorgi 的现象学分析方法和 Colaizzi 的资料分析方法,扎
根理论中 Glaser 和 Strauss 的三级编码分析,以及民族志分析
(ethnographic accounts)、揭露分析(disclosure analysis)和叙事分析
(narrative analysis)。另一类资料分析方法相对独立于具体的理论
和认知论,并且可以广泛应用于不同的质性研究中;这一类分析方法
包括内容分析法(content analysis)和主题分析法(thematic
analysis),以下就这两种方法进一步说明。

1) 内容分析法(content analysis)。

内容分析法具有系统性(systematic)、客观性(objective)和定量
性(quantitative)的特点。内容分析法将收集的资料整理、分类、抽
象、提炼后用文字或图表表达意义,本质上是一种对文本"去粗存精"
的过程(coding scheme),尤其适用于应用 Nvivo 软件进行数据分析。

如示例 4 - 16 所示,作者在资料分析部分的第二段陈述了内容

分析法的步骤包括 4 位研究者独立进行系统编码（systematic coding）、形成初始编码树（initial coding tree）、完善编码树（modified during the analysis process）和使用到的技术包括比较与对比（comparing and contrasting）。第三段描述了具体的翻译与抽象化过程，包括确定模式与主题（identifying patterns and meanings of the themes）及分析描述核心类别、类别及主题。最后，作者还详细描述了确保信息饱和（saturation）的举措。

示例 4 - 16　内容分析法

A content analysis method was used，starting with systematic coding by four independent researchers. The initial coding tree was modified during the analysis process. By comparing and contrasting similar categories across all interviews，emerging themes were inductively derived from the raw data. Finally，categories and sub-categories were organized based on the raw data and theoretical framework（Tong et al.，2007）. The interpretation and abstraction process included identifying patterns and meanings of the themes. The relationships between the core category，main categories，and subcategories were identified and described. Theoretical saturation was achieved when no new insights were identified from the data. Saturation was reached after eight interviews with cardiac rehabilitation participants and ten interviews with community participants. Four more interviews （two in each group） were conducted to ensure saturation. Finally，the findings were discussed and compared to existing literature（Graneheim et al.，2017）.

2）主题分析法(thematic analysis)。

主题分析法被（潜在地）认为是现实（realist）或经验性（experiential）的分析方法,具有灵活性(flexible)与实用性(useful)的特点。由于主题分析非常灵活,常常是很多其他数据分析方法的第一步,所以很多学者并没有把主题分析列为一个单独的分析方法。直到2006年,Braun 和 Clarke 给了主题分析清晰的定义与步骤,主题分析才开始慢慢地在研究方法中有了独立的地位。Braun 和 Clarke 认为"主题(theme)"代表的是数据中出现的元素(essence),而"主题分析(thematic analysis)"就是将这些主题系统再现的过程。Braun 和 Clarke 的主题分析法分为6个步骤。

下面将以示例 4 – 17 为例,进行介绍。此研究的分析问题（analytic question）为"What experiences, perception/s drive the process of nurses' implicit rationing of their care?",围绕这个问题,研究者通过以下步骤来对资料进行分析: ① 熟悉数据(familiarization with the data):对文本反复阅读(reading and rereading the transcripts)。②产生初始编码(initial coding phase):研究者们分别阅读文本并对模式和主题进行编码(coding for patterns and themes),标记相关、有意义的段落(labeling paragraphs that contained information regarding points discussed)。③寻找共同主题(themes):研究者们再次分析初始编码,并将编码分类,形成主题,就主题的含义及涌现的模式进行讨论并达成一致意见(the two analyzed the initial codes together, sorted them into potential themes and discussed their meanings and emerging patterns with the aim of reaching a shared understanding/agreement)。④检查主题:将所有提取的编码信息归入相应主题和思维导图(all relevant coded data extracts were collated within the identified themes and mind-maps),检查所确定主题的内部同质性(internal homogeneity)和外部异质性(external heterogeneity),在必要时对提取的数据进行

再次编码（re-coding）。⑤定义主题（refined and defined the themes）：研究者通过确认主题的个体性和集体性本质（identifying their individual and collective essence），进一步完善和定义这些主题。⑥形成报告：经过以上分析步骤，以及对个体访谈和各个访谈间的归纳性分析，最终形成概念性主题（Conceptual themes were derived inductively from analysis within and between individual interviews）。在数据分析中，作者还应用了 MAXQDA 软件辅助分析。

示例 4-17 主题分析法

A thematic analysis approach was used, following the phases described by Braun and Clarke (Braun and Clarke, 2006). As thematic analysis is very flexible and facilitates distinguishing, identifying, and interpreting themes, i. e., significant patterns in the data, we considered it appropriate for use with interpretive descriptive methodology. Overall, the thematic analysis was guided by one analytic question: What experiences, perception/s drive the process of nurses' implicit rationing of their care? After reading and re-reading the transcripts (familiarization with the data), the initial coding phase started with the first and last authors (*Blinded*) reading the transcripts separately and coding for patterns and themes, labeling paragraphs that contained information regarding points discussed. In the next phase, the two analyzed the initial codes together, sorted them into potential themes and discussed their meanings and emerging patterns with the aim of reaching a shared understanding/agreement.

For the next step, all relevant coded data extracts were collated within the identified themes and mind-maps used to meaningfully organize any emerging themes. The two authors reviewed the identified themes for internal homogeneity (i. e., meaningful cohesion of codes) and external heterogeneity (i. e., clear distinctions between themes), re-coding the data extracts as necessary. They further refined and defined the themes by identifying their individual and collective essence (Braun and Clarke, 2006). Conceptual themes were derived inductively from analysis within and between individual interviews (Hunt, 2009; Thorne, 2008; Thorne et al., 2004). We used MAXQDA 2018 (VERBI Software, 2017) for data analysis.

抛开不同的学派与方法,质性研究的资料分析采用归纳法(inductive),以明确主题和主题间的关系为目标,通过阅读原材料(reading)、编码(coding)、分类(categorizing)、浓缩(condensing)、提炼主题(theme)和(或)本质(essence)来解释现象的实质和意义。形成的主题具有准确性、独立性、互斥性和穷尽性。

5. 伦理学考虑

在质性研究中,伦理学考虑贯穿始终。从研究设计时的确立访谈提纲和问题,到访谈开始前研究对象的招募与告知,以及访谈全程患者对参与研究的自主权,都需要考虑伦理。论文撰写过程中,需要陈述研究的伦理学审查情况(例如,研究是否通过伦理审查、研究中如何保护患者权利)。如示例 4 – 18 所示,该文陈述了伦理相关内

容,包括伦理审查具体单位、知情同意过程中对研究目及自愿原则的
说明、书面知情同意书的获取、保护患者隐私所采取的措施。

示例4－18　伦理学考虑

Approval was granted by the hospital's Helsinki human subjects committee and a college based ethical committee. The study objectives and voluntary nature of the study were explained to participants, who were told they have the right to withdraw from the study at any time. Written informed consent was obtained. Confidentiality was assured by not revealing the identity of the participants.

6. 可信度

质性研究很少使用量性研究中的信度和效度,而是使用"可信度
(trustworthiness)"来描述整个研究结果的严谨性(rigor)。此概念
由 Lincoln 和 Guba 在 1985 年提出,并引入了 4 项衡量质性研究可
信性和严谨性的指标,即可信性（credibility）、可靠性
（dependability）、可确认性（confirmability）和可转移性
（transferability）。可通过不同的方法来实现研究的可信度。

如示例4－19所示。可信性(credibility)通过开展深入访谈(in-depth interview)、同行汇报(peer debriefing)及研究者自身的可信度
来实现。可靠性(dependability)通过过程审查(process audit)来实
现,如详细地记录数据分析的每一步以供同行评阅(documentation
of every step in the analysis process was maintained for evaluation
by peer researchers)。可确认性(confirmability)通过描述决策过程
来实现(Confirmability was established by providing a description

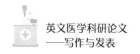
and rationale for the decisions made based on the findings，helping to ensure they accurately portrayed participants' responses）。可转移性(transferability)通过提供足够多的描述性资料来实现，如对深入访谈进行大量（extensive）、丰富（rich）、详细（detailed）的描述，以便他人对资料进行评价。

示例 4 - 19　可信度包含内容

Criteria of credibility，transferability，dependability，and confirmability were used to establish study trustworthiness (Guba and Lincoln，1989）. **Credibility** was achieved by in-depth interviews with participants followed by peer debriefing. The primary investigator performed coding，categorization，and analysis of all the data. **Dependability** was reached by process audit，i. e.，documentation of every step in the analysis process was maintained for evaluation by peer researchers. **Confirmability** was established by providing a description and rationale for the decisions made based on the findings，helping to ensure they accurately portrayed participants' responses. **Transferability** was established by extensive descriptions collected through in-depth interviews. The descriptions provide the basis for outside reviewers to judge transferability (Guba and Lincoln，1989）.

第5节　研究结果

质性研究论文的结果可分为类属型（categorization）或情境型

（contextualization）。前者使用分类的方法，将研究结果按照一定的主题分门别类地陈述，具有较强的逻辑性和层次性；后者注重情境和过程，按照事件发生的时间序列或时间之间的逻辑关联进行描述。目前，护理研究中以类属型的结果汇报方式为主。

在论文撰写时，研究结果部分一般以一段高度总结性的文字来展现。这段文字将发现的主题（themes）以精简的语言串起来，以使读者对研究结果形成一个整体性印象。如示例 4-20 所示，结果部分，第一段总结了研究的现象和主要研究结果；并且使用图片更清晰地展示了研究结果。

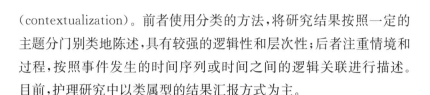

示例 4-20　对结果的概括性描述

In this section, we present our findings on frontline nurses'（IN）and ward nurse managers'（IWM）day-to-day experiences with implicit rationing of nursing care on their units. The fact that rationing occurs reveals a gap between the ideal and the reality of providing nursing care. According to the study participants, implicit rationing occurs when nurses have difficulty maintaining stability in complex situations. At the micro-level, nurses described various strategies they applied to prevent or reduce the need for rationing. Within each theme, we identified subthemes that nurses described as important factors influencing their decision-making, priority setting, and rationing decisions (see **Fig. 1**).

有时，研究者也会采用流程图的形式对研究结果进行立体、系统、清晰的展现。如示例 4-21 所示，作者采用主题图（thematic map）的形式，生动、全面地展示了急诊护士在决策、确定优先事项和

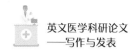
护理配给这一过程中涌现出来的三个主题和亚主题。关于图表的应用及要点，将会在**本章第 7 节**中进一步阐述。

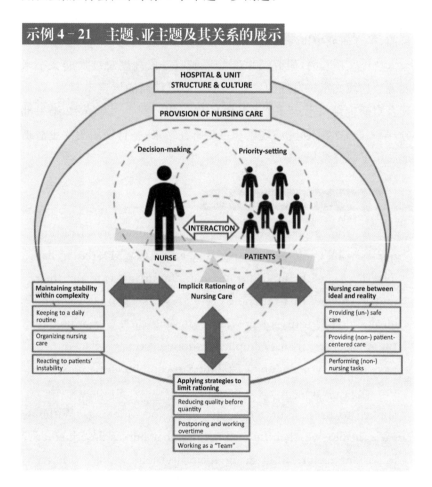

示例 4 - 21　主题、亚主题及其关系的展示

需要注意的是，此处的主题（theme）具有抽象性（abstract）和概括性（generalized），不是研究问题或访谈问题的简单转换或凝练。如示例 4 - 22 所示，研究问题为"护士对急诊医院隐性护理配给的体会（nurses' experiences with implicit rationing of nursing care in acute-care hospitals)"。访谈问题围绕着以下方面开展：一线急诊科护士的隐性护理配给的经验（experiences as frontline nurses/nurse ward managers with implicit rationing of nursing care）、对临床决策和优先次序设定的看法（perceptions regarding clinical decision-making and priority setting）、以及对患者和（或）护理活动优先次序的看法（perspectives on prioritization of patients and/or care activities）。作者将研究结果归纳为 3 个主题，分别是：①在复杂情况下保持稳定（Maintaining stability within complexity）；②运用策略限制配给（Applying strategies to limit rationing）；③理想与现实之间的护理（Nursing care between ideal and reality）。每个主题均包含亚主题（sub-themes），如**第一个主题的亚主题为**：a. 保持日常的生活规律（Keeping to a daily routine）；b. 组织护理工作（Organizing nursing care）；c. 对患者的不稳定因素做出反应（Reacting to patients' instability）。

示例 4-22　研究结果中的主题及亚主题

3.1　Maintaining stability within complexity

Clinical practice in acute-care settings is highly complex. Within the complexity of patient needs, care and work processes, and health care technologies, nurses seek to create and maintain stability within their environment. Stability is supporting by keeping to daily routines that help nurses exert control over their practice, for example by structuring the diverse and often competing demands of their patients and their work environment.

3.1.1　Keeping to a daily routine

In order to maintain stability under complex or otherwise stressful conditions, nurses reported following *a predetermined daily routine* of nursing care (IN2)... One nurse ward manager described how the nurses on her ward adhered to a routine focusing on nursing tasks: *On a normal day we start in the morning by measuring the blood pressure; then we take care of the oral therapy and I start at room 1. If there is nothing special, then I go room by room, from room 1 to 7and then from room 8 to 13（IWM3）.*

结果部分应当有足够的证据资料，强调"深入描述 thick description"。一个好的"结果"能够提供大量、适宜、细节性的原始资料来支撑主题和亚主题[多通过引用（quotes）访谈者的原话来实现]。引用的可以是几段话、一段话、一句话、一个短语或一个单词；用引号标出（不同杂志的格式要求可能不同），并且标注来源（被访者代码、简单特征及访谈轮次等）。当研究结果包含主题和亚主题时（多数质性研究是这样的），主题多为 headings，quotes 则出现在亚主题中。如示例 4 - 22 所示，研究者在亚主题的段落部分，使用斜体来展现 quotes，并在每一个 quotes 后面标注其来源。有的研究者会将 quotes 单独置于一段，以支撑整个或部分亚主题。如示例 4 - 23 所示，斜体部分为受访者的原话，作者将其以独立段落的形式呈现出来，用于支撑亚主题；同时，在段落开始，说明了 quotes 来源。

示例 4 - 23　单独成段的 quotes

3.1.2　Willpower

A theme that was repeatedly articulated by the participants dealt with self-determination. Participants expressed the need for free will in order to be motivated to incorporate modifications in their lifestyle.

67 years（Cardiac rehabilitation） "*It's all about willpower，you shouldn't panic，it's willpower，thinking rationally. I understood that if I will not take care，I will suffer more. I must do something about it. A person must come to the conclusion by himself. Pushing or yelling wouldn't help.*"

最后，值得注意的是，质性研究的主题和亚主题大多以名词或动名词的形式出现。如上文中提到的主题中，使用了名词"nursing care between ideal and reality""adherence facilitators and barriers""willpower"等，动名词"maintaining""applying""keeping""organizing""reacting"等；这些词都充分体现了质性研究主题的概括性和抽象性，也潜在地反映了质性研究的现象是身处其中的个体正在进行的真实生活体验(lived experience)，质性研究结果具有"鲜活性"。

第6节 讨 论

质性研究论文的讨论部分主要包含两部分内容。首先，对本研究的结果和意义进行概括性总结。研究者应对本研究的结果呈现了什么样的社会、文化或实践问题/情境/现象进行陈述，展现出 whole picture of the issue/situation/phenomenon 以及这些问题/情境/现象可能的原因、过程和影响因素；阐释本研究结果与既往类似研究或理论的联系；说明本研究对于相关研究领域的贡献。其次，要与前言部分呼应，再次强调本研究的意义。当然，在讨论的最后，还需要给出结论。

如示例 4 - 24 所示，作者用"The results of our study highlighted the importance of...", "The results described..."等引

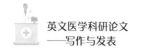

出本研究的意义与结果。

示例 4 - 24　讨论部分引出主要研究结果及意义

The results of our study highlighted the importance of taking the whole person into consideration by focusing on patients' overall life situations and integrating the social，mental and physical aspects of their lives to understand their experience of CRF. **The results described** how oncology nurses were able to achieve a personal relationship of understanding to support the men with CRF.

　　讨论中，需要将本研究结果与既往研究进行对比和分析。这些对比与分析可以是与本研究结果一致的、不同的或有分歧的。如示例 4 - 25 所示，研究者引用既往结果对本研究结果进行支持并分析可能出现此结果的原因。

示例 4 - 25　与既往研究的对比和分析

　　The oncology nurses in this study noted that men with CRF generally avoid talking about their experiences with the condition. *Research*（24）has shown that cancer patients often experience CRF as a new sensation and therefore have difficulty finding the words to describe it. *Studies*（25，26）have demonstrated that fatigue is often an unexpressed symptom and that there is a belief among patients that fatigue has to be managed alone because other people do not want to hear about or understand their condition.

这一部分，还需要对研究的特色（strengths）及局限性和不足之处（limitations）进行讨论。如示例4-26所示，作者分析了研究的特色，包括：①样本量充足：足够大的样本量以确保研究能进行深入分析；②多种数据收集方法以获得丰富的数据：应用半结构式问卷来补充收集资料，丰富质性访谈中相关重要信息。此外，作者还列举了研究的局限性，如样本纳入时未严格遵循纳入标准、结果的外延性不强。需要注意的是，尽管作者列出了研究的局限性，针对每个不足之处，作者均给予了一定的解释（"the rich experience"，"can be transferred to similar situations"）。通过此种方式，说明这些局限性瑕不掩瑜，研究依然具有科学性。

示例4-26　研究的特色及局限性

Study strengths and limitations

This study sought to describe oncology nurses' experiences of meeting with men with cancer and talking about CRF. Nine oncology nurses were recruited using a purposeful sampling method and subsequently participated in the present study. This number was considered sufficient to maintain depth in the analysis and offered an excellent opportunity to study the various experiences of oncology nurses. The sample size in qualitative research should be large enough to achieve variations in experiences yet small enough to permit a deep analysis of the data (32). A further strength of this study was the rich data collected using questions that followed a semi-structured interview guide. The shortest interview lasted 30 minutes but was substantial as it contributed and complemented the other interviews with important data.

The study also had limitations. For example, one of the participants had worked as an oncology nurse for a shorter period than stipulated in the inclusion criteria, which required participants to have had at least three years' experience as an oncology nurse in municipal health care. This participant was motivated for their participation based on the rich experience of meeting with men with CRF. Finally, the results of this study cannot be generalised, but they can be transferred to similar situations (13).

此部分,亦可讨论研究对护理实践、研究、教育、管理等领域的建议与启示(implications),如示例 4-27 所示。当然,根据期刊不同,这些内容也可放在结论部分。

示例 4-27 本研究对未来实践的启示

This observation indicates the importance of making experiences of cancer-related fatigue visible. Oncology nurses therefore have a responsibility to ask about cancer-related fatigue and to make the men in their care aware of the symptom. Increased patient knowledge of this condition can support oncology nurses as they attempt to facilitate individual fatigue management among men.

与量性研究论文类似,质性研究论文的最后,也需要给出相应的总结。该总结是对研究核心内容的高度凝练(包括内容和结果)。如示例 4-28 所示,该总结中,作者再次回到研究目的,简述了研究内容,并对结果中得出的主题进行汇总。此外,作者还在这里提到了本

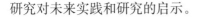

研究对未来实践和研究的启示。

示例 4 - 28　总结举例

Based on the perspectives of people living with dementia, their informal caregivers and healthcare professionals, we can conclude that to empower a person living with dementia, it is important that they have a sense of personal identity, can make their own choices, that their capabilities are addressed, and that they can experience a sense of worth. The four themes of empowerment seem to be important both at home and in nursing homes, and in different stages of dementia. However, support must be adjusted to the personal situation and individual capabilities, and, therefore, practical detailing of support differs. Our empowerment framework provides a basis for developing interventions to empower people living with dementia and to support（in）formal caregivers in this empowerment process.

第 7 节　其他要点

　　不同于量性研究,质性研究论文对于图表的应用没有那么频繁和复杂。通常为简单的三线表或流程图,多出现在研究方法或结果部分。

　　在研究方法部分,如果研究采用了半结构式访谈法收集资料,研究者可以列表举例访谈提纲中涉及的问题及提词,如示例 4 - 29 所示。

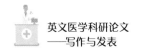

英文医学科研论文
——写作与发表

示例 4 - 29 列表展示访谈提纲

Topic	Questions and prompts
About you	• Q. Could you tell me about your current pregnancy status and tell me a bit about how your pregnancy has been so far? Prompt：What stage are you at in your pregnancy/post-pregnancy? • Q. How would you describe your PA levels? Prompt：What did you expect your PA levels to be like once you got pregnant? Prompt：Did your PA change between trimesters?
Views on PA during pregnancy	• Q. What are your thoughts on PA during pregnancy? Prompt：Do you think it is safe/risky?
Costs and benefits of PA	• Q. What are your views of the costs and benefits of doing PA whilst pregnant? Prompt：Do you feel the costs outweigh the benefits/benefits outweigh the costs?

　　有时,研究者为了展现数据分析的可靠性,或使读者更清楚地了解数据是如何一步一步分析的,也会采用图表的形式展现数据分析过程。如示例 4 - 30 所示。

示例4-30 图表展示数据分析过程

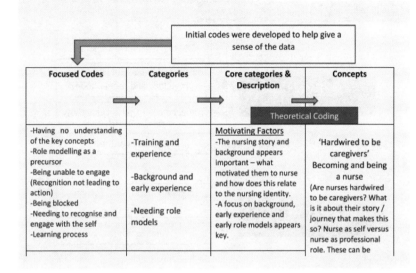

在研究结果部分,图表的使用更为常见。如,可用简单"一对一"的表格来展示研究对象的一般性特征或情景性特征(如上文所述)。有时,也会对研究对象进行简单的统计描述,便于读者对研究对象的一般情况有所了解,增加研究的可信度和可靠性。质性研究中的图表也可以更直观、系统、简明地展示研究结果——主题(themes)、亚主题(subthemes),有时可以包含类别(categories)及代表性编码(codes),如示例4-31和示例4-32所示。

示例4-31 使用表格展示研究结果

Overview of codes, categories and themes.

Themes (heading) and categories	Codes
Having a sense of personal identity	
Being the person you have always been	*Know the person: life history and habits*
Being the person you are now	*Know the person: wishes and needs*
Having a sense of choice and control	
Making own choices	*Making your own choices, freedom in choices*
Choices are accepted and respected	*Accept choice of person living with dementia, nothing is mandatory*
Making choices is supported when needed	*Maintain autonomy with support*
Having a sense of usefulness and being needed	
Doing what you can, want, and are used to for as long as possible	*Don't take over tasks, start with new habits in good time*
Being activated and challenged	*Involve person living with dementia in daily tasks, try what activates someone*
Retaining a sense of worth	
Feeling valued	*Retain sense of worth, dignity*
Being heard and seen	*Talk to the person living with dementia*
Participating in society	*Dementia-friendly society, knowledge about dementia*

示例 4 - 32　使用图展示研究结果

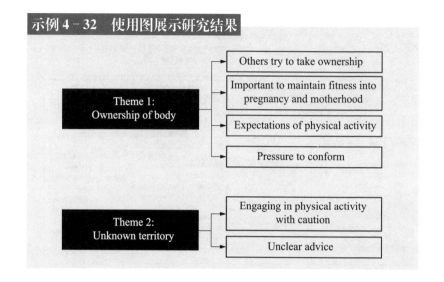

　　与量性研究的图表使用目的一致,质性研究中图表同样是对文字的立体浓缩,可更加清楚、生动、系统地展现出资料所蕴含的各种信息、意义和联系。研究者可以根据自己的研究设计及资料特点,选择适宜的形式对资料进行归类与展示。在设计图表时,需要考虑:这个图表是否可以清楚地展现我所采用的数据收集(或分析)方法?是否清楚地展示我所找到的数据资料?资料之间的关系是否展示清楚?图表设计其实是一个思考的过程,可以帮助研究者理清思路,把握核心问题,更加清楚地展现研究成果。

第5章 系统文献综述撰写要点

循证医学使用现有的医学证据来指导临床决策并对临床建议的强度进行评估。在临床实践中,医学人员根据指南推荐,对患者的诊断和治疗方案进行选择。系统文献综述对现阶段研究结果进行系统、严格的评估和整合,其所产生的证据是制定指南时的重要参考资源。本章对系统文献综述的常见类型及撰写要点进行详细介绍,将回答以下几个问题。

- 系统文献综述有哪些常见类型?
- 如何撰写一个完整有吸引力的标题和摘要?
- 如何构建简洁明了、有逻辑的前言和(或)背景?
- 系统文献综述的方法部分有哪些注意事项?
- 撰写系统文献综述应该避免哪些常见错误?
- 撰写系统文献综述前应完成哪些准备工作?
- 汇报系统文献综述时应涵盖哪些要点?

第1节 系统文献综述类型

1. 系统文献综述的概念

作为各类文献综述的"金标准",系统文献综述是针对某个研究问题,通过运用系统、科学、严谨的方法,全面地收集、评价及整合现阶段相关研究证据。Petticrew & Roberts 将系统文献综述定义为"A review that strives to comprehensively identify, appraise, and synthesize all the relevant studies on a given topic using methods that are well-defined and clearly reported"。

系统文献综述具有以下价值:①研究结论基于既往多项研究,考虑各研究的偏倚,所产生的结果可能更加准确和可信;②识别出各研究间存在的异质性及其来源;③通过对各研究进行横向对比,发现潜在的影响因素;④识别现阶段研究存在的局限性及空缺处(research gap);⑤是促进临床实践和制定政策的有效方法。

系统文献综述中常见的一些问题:①"apples and oranges":各个研究差异太大,以至于无法进行有意义的综合性分析;②"garbage in and garbage out":所选文献质量太差,最后得出的结果不可信;③"sloppy thinking":思维、方法马虎、不严谨;④"reductionist":过度简化,无法反映证据的复杂性和细微差别。

如何预防以上问题:①避免选择太宽泛的主题;②开展文献回顾时,考虑原始文献的质量;③严格遵循系统文献回顾的方法;④对于无法进行量化的结果,采用定性的分析方法。

作为学生及青年学者,为何要考虑开展文献综述? ①低风险/高收益(性价比高):低风险,可控性强,较少受到外界因素干扰(例如,疫情期间,无法开展相关研究);一般都能够发表出去(不管结果是否是阳性)。高收益,与单独的原始研究相比,更容易受到关注、被引用。②进行文献综述这一研究过程,本身是有益的:通过检索文献,有利于你与本领域其他学者取得联系;通过阅读其他人的研究,提升你对该领域知识的积累并加深你对某研究方法的认识;通过与团队其他成员的密切联系,建立良好的合作基础;还可以强化评判性思维。③文献综述对于个人时间上的付出需求较大,对于外界资源的需求较少,这对于学生及处于职业生涯初期的研究人员来说,十分重要。

2. 系统文献综述常见类型

综述的类型有很多种,范围最广的是"文献综述"(literature review)。此种综述是对现阶段文献的回顾和分析,多数情况下未进行系统性的检索。所以,其所包含文献的全面性及结果的准确性无法得到保障。相比而言,系统文献综述在方法学上更加严谨。如果系统文献综述中,可对各研究间的数据进行量化,则可开展 meta-analysis。图 5 - 1 展示了综述、系统文献综述和 meta-analysis 之间的关系。

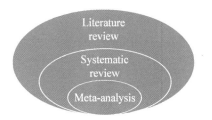

图 5 - 1 综述类型介绍

对于系统文献综述,常见的两大类包括无法进行量化的 systematic review 和可以进行量化的 meta-analysis;其他类型还包括 integrative review、scoping review、umbrella review、state-of-the-art review。下面,将着重对**系统文献综述**所包含的主要类型进行简介。

Systematic review 的主要目的是针对某个研究问题系统性地回顾、评价及汇总相关证据。该方法采用定性的方法对来自各个研究的主要发现进行汇总,不会用到统计分析方法。在使用该方法时,各研究结果主要以表格的形式呈现出来,并结合文字进行描述。

Meta-analysis 的主要目的是提供一个较明确的效应值（effect size）。该综述在 systematic review 的基础上，采用定量的方法对各个研究中的数据进行汇总，需要使用到统计分析方法。在使用该方法时，各研究结果（包括 95% 可信区间）及汇总结果主要以森林图的形式呈现。森林图中，各研究根据样本量的不同所占权重不同；图中还可展示各研究间存在的异质性大小。通过 meta-analysis，读者针对某研究问题，可以获得一个量化效应值。

Integrative review 是一种综合性文献综述，对既往理论性和实证性文献进行回顾和整合，进而为某特定现象或健康问题提供更加全面的了解。此综述范围广，可以纳入不同类型的研究（描述性或实验性）；目的较宽泛（例如：确定某概念的定义、对某理论进行回顾、对方法学进行汇总分析）。此方法在**护理领域**中应用较广泛，可参考 Whittemore 和 Knafl 提出的方法学开展。

Scoping review 是一个相对较新的系统文献综述类型，回答探索性的研究问题。"Scoping reviews are useful for examining emerging evidence when it is still unclear what other, more specific questions can be posed and valuably addressed by a more precise systematic review"，可视为 systematic review 的前身。其主要目的是通过回顾现阶段相关研究涉及的文献范围（scope or coverage of a body of literature：）、证据类型（type of evidence, e. g., overview, summary, policy papers）、核心概念（key concept and related factors）及研究方法（how research is conducted, e. g., methodology），为未来的重点研究方向提供证据。例如，如果综述的目的是了解目前所有测量睡眠的便携式设备的准确性，则可采用是 scoping review 这种方法。该类综述也涉及系统、完整的文献检索，可纳入正在进行的研究；无须对纳入的文献进行质量评价。

Umbrella review 是对已有综述的综述（synthesis of existing reviews），此方法使作者可以对不同综述之间的异同点进行比较。

其一大特点是：多纳入证据水平较高的文献（即：systematic review and meta-analysis）。此方法的目的不是重复数据库检索、评估研究质量或对纳入的综述结果进行评估，而是针对某个特定的研究问题，对既往综述的发现进行总结。例如，单个系统文献综述可以是检验某特定干预措施的有效性；但是，umbrella review 可以对不同干预措施的效果进行总结。因此，此类综述能够为临床决策者提供更加全面和直观的信息，更有利于临床实践和制定相关政策。针对如何开展 umbrella review，Joanna Briggs Institute 提出了初步指南，可供参考。

State-of-the-art review 是对某领域最新的研究进展进行综述，以寻找研究趋势、一致点和争议点。对于刚接触该领域的人或想要发现潜在研究方向的人来说，此类综述具有较大的阅读价值。因为人们仅从此类综述中，便可找到研究前沿趋势。由于受到时效性的影响，此类综述可能无法为某领域的研究进展提供全面的描述。一般情况下，多是对某领域十分熟悉的专家（权威）开展此类综述。

现对以上几种常见类型的系统文献综述所具备的特点进行总结，如表 5－1 所示。在众多文献综述类型中，systematic review and meta-analysis 是最常见的，其在撰写的方法学上也是涵盖面相对较广的。因此，本章节将着重对此类综述的撰写进行介绍。

表 5－1　不同类型系统文献综述比较

类型	综述方案（protocol）	系统、完整的检索	文献质量评价	数据整合	分析重点
System review	是	是	是	文字描述结合表格	已知的、未知的、不确定的，对未来研究和实践的建议
Meta-analysis	是	是	是	图表为主，文字补充	对效应大小进行量化

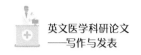
（续表）

类型	综述方案（protocol）	系统、完整的检索	文献质量评价	数据整合	分析重点
Integra-tive review	是（非必须）	是	是	文字描述结合表格	全面了解某主题，总结理论性和实证性证据
Scoping review	是（非必须）	是：受时间段和范围限制	否	表格为主，文字补充	根据文献范围、类型等对文献数量和质量进行描述
Umbrella review	是	是：对综述进行检索	是	图表为主，文字补充	已知的、未知的、对未来研究和实践的建议
State-of-the-art review	否	是：以当代文献为主	否	文字为主，表格辅助	现阶段围绕某领域的知识现况，未来研究重点

第2节　标题和摘要

　　与其他类型的论文类似，标题和摘要的重要性不言而喻。本书**第2章**对标题和摘要的撰写要点进行了详细介绍，这里仅补充一下对于综述来说比较有特色的撰写要点。

1. 标题

　　标题需要体现研究涉及的核心内容（例如，研究人群），可以参考PICOS（Population，Intervention，Comparison，Outcomes，Study design）或PECO（Population，Exposure，Comparator，Outcomes）的结构书写。需要注意：几乎无一例外，**综述的标题要体现具体的**

设计(即文献类型)。在撰写时,多采用"冒号"+"设计"的形式;有些作者还选择在标题中体现出所纳入文献的类型(例如,systematic review of RCT),如示例 5 - 1 和示例 5 - 2 所示。当然,还有一些标题,首先体现了研究设计,如示例 5 - 3 所示。

示例 5 - 1　标题举例 1

Types of interventions targeting dietary, physical activity，and weight-related outcomes among university students：**A systematic review** of *systematic reviews*

示例 5 - 2　标题举例 2

The effect of a Mediterranean diet on metabolic parameters in patients with non-alcoholic fatty liver disease：**A systematic review** of *randomized controlled trials*

示例 5 - 3　标题举例 3

A **systematic review** of the accuracy of sleep wearable devices for estimating sleep onset

撰写标题没有对错之分,好的标题能够更好地吸引读者。不管采用何种形式,标题均需要体现论文的核心内容和特色。类似于撰写其他类型的论文:有些期刊对于标题的字数有限制,在投稿前,需进行核查;还可下载目标期刊最近发表的文献综述,对比一下自己的标题和该刊近期所接收论文的标题在格式上是否一致。此外,撰写标题时,单词大小写的书写上也有需要遵循的原则,具体可参考**第 2 章第 1 节**。

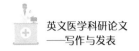
2. 摘要

摘要的目的是使读者知道：研究做了什么？怎么做？发现了什么？研究结果有何启示？同标题一样，摘要的内容需要简短而丰富。一般情况下，字数在 200～300 字（因期刊而不同）。不可在摘要中使用引文，减少缩写的使用（有些期刊，不允许在摘要中使用缩写）。一般情况下，摘要会留到最后再写。摘要的格式可以分为**结构式摘要和非结构式摘要**。这两种类型的摘要撰写方法，具体细节可参考**第 2章第 1 节**。这里仅对需要格外注意的要点进行介绍。

摘要中能够提供信息的多少，取决于期刊对于摘要字数的要求。但不论字数限制是多少，**结构式摘要均需包含研究背景/目的、方法、结果和结论**。如示例 5 - 4 所示，作者首先介绍了研究背景和目的；继而给出了具体的方法（包括：检索的数据库、涵盖时间、纳入的研究类型）；接着，简要介绍了本研究的主要发现；最后，给出相应的结论和对未来研究的建议。注意：这个摘要的结果中，作者未给出具体的数据（有些期刊要求，不能在结果中给出具体的统计值，例如 P值）。在撰写摘要时，要尤其注意这一点。

示例 5 - 4　结构式摘要举例 1

Background：Dietary habit can play a key role in the prevention and treatment of fatty liver disease (NAFLD). Although many studies have investigated the effect of Mediterranean diet on NAFD, findings are inconsistent and there is no systematic review on this topic. Therefore, the aim of this systematic review is to summarize the effect of Mediterranean diet on serum metabolic indices and anthropometric measures among NAFLD patients.

Methods：We searched titles，abstracts，and keywords of articles indexed in Science Direct，MEDLINE，and Google Scholar databases up to October 2018 to identify eligible RCT studies. Randomized clinical trials assessing the effects of MD on NAFLD were included.

Results：The present study included 10 randomized controlled trials，which involved a total of 856 adults with NAFLD. According to the result，MD may improve anthropometric measures，lipid profile. Glycemic indices，liver enzyme，and NAFLD severity indices among patients with NAFLD.

Conclusion：We found that MD could alleviate NAFLD severity parameters but differences between studies should be taken into account. Finally，in order to draw a firm link between MD and NAFLD，more clinical trials with adequate sample size and better methodology should be done.

再如示例 5 - 5 所示，本摘要中，作者给出了详细的方法，包括检索的数据库、论文类型、时间段、纳入和排除标准、统计分析方法及 PROSPERO 注册号。在结果中，提供了具体的数据（包括效应值、可信区间等）。

示例 5 - 5　结构式摘要举例 2

Methods In this systematic review and meta-analysis，we searched MEDLINE，Embase，the Cochrane Library，and Google Scholar databases for observational studies，systematic reviews，and randomised controlled trials published between Jan 1,2001，and March 31,2017，without language restrictions.

We included studies reporting mortality outcomes for international migrants of any age residing outside their country of birth... We calculated summary estimates using random-effects models. This study is registered with PROSPERO, number CRD42017073608.

Findings Of the 12480 articles identified by our search, 96 studies were eligible for inclusion... The summary estimate of all-cause SMR for international migrants was lower than one when compared with the general population in destination countries (0-70[95% CI 0-65-0-76]; P2=99-8%)... Point estimates of all-cause age-standardized mortality in migrants ranged from 420 to 874 per 100 000 population.

非结构式摘要虽然没有提供明确的小标题,但需要涵盖的核心内容与结构式摘要相同。如示例5-6所示,作者在摘要中给出了研究背景、目的、方法、结果及结论。

示例5-6 非结构式摘要

The pathological use of the internet-conceptualized as 'internet addiction'-might be crucial in initiating and increasing sleep disturbances in the community. While inconsistent evidence is reported regarding the association of internet addiction and sleep disturbances, the severity of this association remains unclear. 【背景】This systematic review and meta-analysis were conducted to increase our understanding of the relationship between internet addiction and sleep disturbances. 【目的】A systematic review was conducted through Scopus, PubMed Central, ProQuest, ISI Web of Knowledge, and EMBASE using key-words related to internet addiction and sleep problems. Observational studies (cohort, case-control, or cross-sectional studies) focusing on association between internet addiction and sleep disturbances including sleep problems and sleep duration were selected. A meta-analysis using random-effect model was conducted to calculate the odds ratio (OR) for experiencing sleep problems and standardized mean differences (SMDs) for sleep duration. 【方法】Eligible studies (N=23) included 35,684 participants. The overall pooled OR of having sleep problems if addicted to the internet was 2.20 (95% CI: 1.77 - 2.74). Additionally, the overall pooled SMDs for sleep duration for the IA group compared to normal internet users was −0.24 (95% CI: −0.38, −0.10). 【结果】Results of the meta-analysis revealed a significant OR for sleep problems and significantly reduced sleep duration among individuals addicted to the internet. 【结论】

　　根据以上内容,在撰写摘要时,提出以下建议:①在撰写"方法"时,可以给出检索的数据库、文献涵盖时间段、纳入的文献类型、主要分析方法(量性的数据统计分析方法或质性的总结方法)、综述注册号。②在撰写"结果"时,对纳入的文献数量进行汇报,对能够反映研究目的的主要结果进行总结。

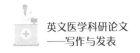
3. 关键词及 Highlight

对于综述的关键词和 highlight，其撰写要点与撰写其他论文类似。具体可以参考**第 2 章第 1 节**。

第 3 节 前 言

与撰写其他类型的论文类似，这里也许要提供相关信息，使读者了解本综述开展的大背景及原因。前言中，需要对本综述相关的文献进行回顾、分析和总结，进而说明本领域未知或需要进一步探索的地方，最后引出所要开展的综述内容，说明该综述如何填补现阶段知识的未知点。值得一提的是，在撰写综述的前言时，一定要对既往已经存在的类似综述进行回顾和总结，进而说明开展本综述的必要性和重要性。

这里，也会涉及一些常见的术语，例如研究问题（research question），研究目的或研究目标（research aim or objective）。本书的**第 2 章第 2 节**对这几个术语的联系和区别进行了详细介绍，可供参考。此外，第 2 章中介绍的撰写技巧，这里也适用。接下来，将通过几个具体示例进行详细说明。

下面，将以一篇发表在 *Sleep Med Rev* 的系统文献综述为例进行详细介绍（这里仅截取了每个短段落的统领句，topic sentence）。本研究的目的是："调查分析成瘾与睡眠障碍的相关性"（This systematic review and meta-analysis were conducted to increase our understanding of the relationship between internet addiction and sleep disturbances）。在研究背景中，**第一段**说明了"近年来，网络的普及性"（Internet use has grown significantly in recent decades）；第

二段引出了本研究的主要内容"网络成瘾这一问题的普遍性"
[Pathological or compulsive use of the internet (often
conceptualized as 'internet addiction') has an inconsistent
prevalence among different populations];第三段和第四段澄清了
"网络成瘾的特点"及"带来的不良后果"(Excessive use of the
internet comprises problematic behavior in human interactions with
information and communication technologies, and has become a
major public health problem);第五段以一篇既往的文献综述开头,
说明了"网络成瘾与精神、心理健康的关系"(In a systematic review,
Carli et al. [6] reported the association between pathological internet
use and related psychopathology),同时引出了睡眠障碍这一主要内
容;第六段中,具体说明了现阶段关于"网络成瘾与睡眠障碍相关性"
的研究进展(The excessive use of social media and internet plays an
important role in initiating and increasing sleep disturbances within
the younger community),这一段也是本研究背景中的核心段落,这
里将对其展开介绍(如示例 5 - 7 所示)。首先,作者回顾了既往原创
性研究结果,发现各个研究的结果均不一致。紧接着,引出了 2014
年发表的一篇文献综述。在肯定这篇综述的同时,也提出了其可进
一步完善的地方;进而顺理成章地引出**最后一段**。

示例 5 - 7 研究背景第六段

The excessive use of social media and internet plays an
important role in initiating and increasing sleep disturbances
within the younger community[43]. ***De Vries et al. found that***
internet users with psychiatric disorders are more likely to
experience sleep problems, depression, anxiety, and
autism[20]. ***Several studies*** have considered the quality of sleep
in people with IA[12,18,44-46], but in some studies no significant

relationship has been found[19]. In studies that have reported a significant relationship between IA and sleep disturbances, the severity of such a relationship has been varied. For example, Kiatzawa et al. reported that university students with problematic internet use reported 52% higher chance of sleeping disturbances than those with ordinary internet use[45], while Li et al. reported that the chance of having sleep problems in students with IA was three times higher than in normal internet users[47]. *A systematic review in 2014 reported* an association between online gaming addiction, problematic internet use (PIU), and sleep problems. The results of the study showed that pathological internet use appeared to be associated with a low sleep quality and subjective insomnia[18]. *Although this study provided valuable information* concerning the relationship between internet use and sleep disturbances, *a quantitative meta-analysis of findings has never been conducted on this relationship and the severity of the association remains unclear.*

　　在本研究背景的最后一段，作者提出了开展本综述的重要性、必要性以及研究目的。如示例 5-8 所示。

示例 5-8　研究背景最后一段

Considering the importance of IA and its potentially increasing prevalence, further studies are needed to examine related factors and negative consequences. Despite the increasing number of studies on this field, ***there has been no recent review*** examining the relationship between IA and sleep disturbances. Therefore, ***to summarize*** available findings and ***collate*** more solid evidence ***for a deeper understanding*** of the relationship between IA and sleep disturbances, the present systematic review and meta-analysis was conducted.

再以另一篇文献综述为例[这里仅截取了每个段落的统领句（topic sentence）]，本研究的目的是："调查地中海饮食在非酒精脂肪肝患者中的效果"（the aim of this systematic review is to summarize the effect of Mediterranean diet on serum metabolic indices and anthropometric measures among non-alcoholic fatty liver disease patients）。

第一段，作者对"非酒精脂肪肝"进行了概述（包括定义、患病率、机制、治疗）（Non-alcoholic fatty liver disease is defined as an increased accumulation of triglyceride in hepatocyte either due to increased inflow of free fatty acids or de novo hepatic lipogenesis）；第二段，提出了"治疗性饮食对非酒精脂肪肝的作用"[Over the past decades, several therapeutic diets including dietary approaches to stop hypertension（DASH）, Ornish, Atkins, the vegetarian-based and Mediterranean diet（MD）have been investigated in the prevention or treatment of NAFLD]，并着重介绍了地中海饮食；第三段，介绍了"目前关于地中海饮食对非酒精脂肪肝的效果"；最后一段，总结并解释了"现阶段研究结果不一致的原因"，进而引出了开展本综述的原因及内容（Studies that assessed the effects of MD on NAFLD have controversies. These studies used different methods for assessing NAFLD severity and also in different populations.

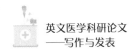
Moreover，relatively small sample size has been used in the majority of the studies assessing this efficacy. To address these issues，we carried out this systematic review by pooling the results from Randomized clinical trials（RCT）studies to examine the effectiveness of MD in the treatment of NAFLD among the adult population. ）

第4节 研究方法

系统文献综述的研究方法，也有特定的写作模式。这一部分需要体现：研究设计（method）、检索方法（search strategy）、纳入和排除标准（inclusion and exclusion criteria）、文献选择步骤（study selection）、数据提取方法（data extraction）、质量评价方法（quality appraisal）和数据分析方法（data synthesis or analysis）。撰写这一部分时，需要遵守的一大原则是，给出完整的细节，以确保其他研究人员可以根据你所提供的信息，对本综述进行复制。

1. 研究设计

在介绍研究设计时，需要说明综述的开展遵守了哪些指南，常见的是 Cochrane 的 Preferred Reporting Items for Systematic Reviews and Meta-Analyses（PRISMA）指南。如果对综述方案进行了注册，还需要提供**注册号**。

多数作者在正式开展文献综述前，会撰写一个初步的方案（类似于科研课题的开题报告），涵盖综述的主要目的和开展方法。系统文献综述可以针对健康问题，提供最佳证据。与基础研究一样，综述的开展也遵循一个系统的研究方法（例如，预先设定的实施方案和分析方法）。但事实上,有些系统文献综述并没有预先制订方案。在没有方案指导的情况下,研究过程中就容易带入偏倚。因此,有必要在开展系统综述前,制订一个文献综述方案。该举措具有至少有 4 个作用(图 5 - 2):①指导作者以防止其做出武断的决定;②思考并记录预先设定好的方法;③如果该方案被发表,可帮助识别出"选择性汇报";④如果该方案被发表,可为其他作者提供参考,防止重复开展类似的综述,也可促进合作。

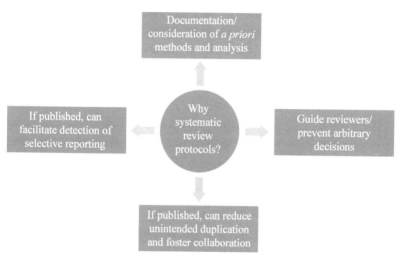

图 5 - 2　制订文献综述方案的 4 个作用

　　在撰写方案时,使用较广泛的是 PROSPERO 数据库所提出的要求,详见相关网站:https://www.crd.york.ac.uk/PROSPERO/。该数据库于 2011 年开始投入使用,用于注册还未开展的系统文献综述,涵盖卫生健康、社会福利、教育、司法和国际发展等领域。虽然不是必须,但是越来越多的期刊都要求作者提供综述的 PROSPERO 注册号。注册提高了综述开展的透明性,不管该综述最终是否被发表,对其方案进行注册有利于减少发表偏倚。如果综述最终被发表,读者还可以通过对比所发表的综述中与注册方案中所汇报的方法,

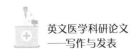
看看二者之间是否存在差异，这有助于防止报告偏见、提高综述质量，并使结果更加可信。

在 PROSPERO 中进行注册时，需要提交该综述相关的目的、方法等关键信息。这些信息被提交以后，会有相关专家进行审查，但不涉及质量评价或同行评议。被审核通过的方案会有一个唯一的注册号，并被发布在公共电子平台。如果综述方案需要进一步完善或作者自己提出变更，可以修改注册信息。同样地，修改过的版本也会发布在此 PROSPERO 电子平台，并在公共记录中显示修改记录。注册记录是永久的，注册人需要提供后续报告和所发表论文相对应的链接。

2. 伦理审查(Ethical Approval)

系统文献综述是对既往文献的回顾和再分析，不涉及直接接触研究对象。因此，无须进行伦理审查及获取知情同意。一般情况下，可以这样写：

Ethical approval and informed consent are not required，as the study will be a literature review and will not involve direct contact with patients(或)Ethical approval is not needed as it is a systematic review of published literature.

3. 检索方法

这一部分可以根据预先注册的方案进行相应的扩展。一般情况下，需要包含检索的数据库，使用的检索词，检索语法(即：如何使用逻辑词将各检索词连接起来)、检索词放在哪里(如，title、abstract、text)。还需说明是否检索了其他来源，例如：灰色文献，相关综述的参考文献，或 ancestry searching(即：对纳入研究的参考文献进行检索），如示例 5 - 9 所示。

示例 5 - 9   文献选择流程

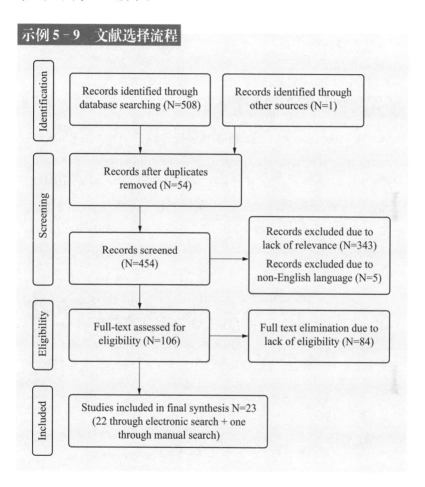

4. 纳入和排除标准

因为每个人的写作风格不一样，纳入和排除标准的撰写存在差异。有一些作者，习惯按照 PICOS 的格式展示；另有一些作者会按照标准的主次进行展示。不管何种方法，所提供的内容都需要科学、清晰、完整。下面将通过一个例子具体说明。如示例 5-10 所示,该文的纳入和排除标准体现了 PICOS 涉及的内容:Population(人群),Intervention(干预),Comparison(对照),Outcomes(结局指标),Study design(研究设计)。

示例 5-10　纳入和排除标准

We included observational (cohort and cross-sectional), systematic reviews, and randomized controlled trials【研究设计】reporting quantitative data on mortality in international migrants of any age residing outside their country of birth【纳入人群】. We excluded studies that recruited participants exclusively from intensive care or high dependency hospital units, with an existing health condition or status (eg, myocardial infarction, HIV, tuberculosis, pregnancy), or a particular health exposure (eg, smoking, high blood pressure)【排除人群】. We also excluded studies limited to maternal or perinatal outcomes.【结局指标】

5. 文献选择

具体如何对文献进行筛选,Cochrane 等指南提供了详细的说明。这里仅从撰写论文的角度出发,提出需要注意的事项。文献的选择过程,可以通过 PRISMA 流程图的形式展示,详见相关网站:http://www.prisma-statement.org/PRISMAStatement/FlowDiagram。流 程 图中,需要体现每个步骤排除了多少篇文献以及排除这些文献的原因。在"Identification"这一步,需要说明通过数据库检索和其他来源分别找到了多少篇文献。目前多数人都通过电子数据库进行检索,且将检索到的文献使用 Endnote 等软件进行文献管理。不同数据库所包含的文献都有交叉,在检索完成后,往往会发现有重复文献。Endnote 软件自带"查重"功能,通过使用此功能,可以较容易地找到重复文献。但是,此方法并不能找到全部的重复文献,需要结合手工查找。当去除重复文献后,可以通过阅读剩余文献的标题和摘要对其进行筛查。筛查的时候,需要参考预先设定好的纳入和排除标准,并对其做好记录。对于初步符合纳入标准的文献,需要进一步获取全文,通过阅读全文进一步进行筛选,确定最终纳入分析的文献数量。如果综述会进行 meta-analysis,流程图中还需说明最终纳入 meta-analysis 的文献数量。

在撰写这一部分时,需要:①说明文献筛选由几个人开展,是否独立开展? ②如果是多人开展,若存在意见不一致的时候,如何去处理? ③无须对"流程图"中的所有信息和数据进行描述,给出核心内容即可。如示例 5 - 11 所示。

示例 5 - 11　文献选择过程中意见不一致时的处理方法

Discrepancies in the inclusion or exclusion of papers during screening were discussed until consensus was achieved, and RWA resolved any final discrepancies.

6. 数据提取

多数情况下,在开始正式的数据提取之前,会预先指定一个数据提取方案(protocol),即表格的"**表头**"(可采用 Word,也可采用 Excel)。该方案可以指导作者在数据提取阶段需要重点提取哪些数

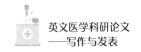
据。常见需要提取的数据包括：研究相关基本信息、研究对象相关信息，以及研究核心方法和主要结果。研究相关基本信息包括：作者(第一作者)、年份、国家、研究设计、样本量。研究对象相关信息例如：年龄、性别、BMI、病程等(如果有的话)。研究核心方法及主要结果包括：主要变量测量方法、干预方案、随访时间、主要结果。此数据提取方案多由文献回顾小组共同决定，并通过在一两篇文献中进行预试验，对此进行相应的调整。形成一个完整的数据提取方案，可大大加速后续工作进程。示例 5 - 12 展示了某文献综述中提取的主要数据；表格下方对表格中使用到的缩写进行了标注。

示例 5 - 12　数据提取表头及编码的使用

Author，year，country	Properzi (30)，2018，Australia
Subjects and gender	F/M：25/26 Both：51
Age range (y) or mean (SD)	51(13.4)
Study design	RCT，parallel
Duration	3-month
Intervention	MD
Dietary assessment	Modified-Burke diet history review
Control	LF diet
Results	Ad libitum diet and MD diets both reduce weight...
Quality score	3

MD：Mediterranean diet，LF：low fat，F：female，M：male；RCT：randomized clinical trial，SD：standard deviation.

在进行数据提取时,要擅长使用编码(coding)。例如,针对"研究设计"这一栏目,纳入综述的各个研究可能采用了不同的研究设计,包括:随机对照试验(RCT)、横断面调查(cross-sectional)或病例对照(case-control)。在表格中,可以采用不同的编码(或缩写)来代表不同的研究设计;同时,在表格下方进行相应的说明。例如,1 表示随机对照试验;2 表示横断面调查;3 表示病例对照。采用此种方法,可以大大缩减表格的篇幅,具有事半功倍的效果。如示例 5 - 12 所示,本综述中,对于性别(女性 F、男性 M)使用了缩写代替;类似地,对于干预措施也采用了缩写表述。同时,在表格的下方,使用了标注进行解释。

对于主要研究结果,需要说明提取的数据格式是怎样的。针对连续性变量,多提取均值和标准差;针对分类变量,多提取频数和百分比。对于有干预的研究,需要说明提取的是干预后数据还是干预前后的差值。如果主要观察指标是相关系数,可以提取相关系数及可信区间;如果主要观察指标是优势比,可以提取 OR 值及可信区间。针对文中的主要研究结果,如果作者未进行汇报(缺失值)或所汇报的内容不符合数据提取格式,需要说明如何处理这种情况。同时,在表格下方,使用标注的形式,说明哪些数据是间接计算来的。如示例 5 - 13 所示,本综述中,对于缺失值,该作者通过文中提供的其他数据计算而来。如示例 5 - 14 所示,本综述中,对于缺失值,该作者通过邮件联系原文作者而获取。类似地,如示例 5 - 15 所示,本综述中,对于缺失值,从图中提取而来。Cochrane 手册中详细地介绍了如何处理缺失值,可进行参考。

示例 5 - 13 缺失值处理方法——根据已有数据计算而来

To assess association between IA and sleep problems, data of 2 * 2 tables calculating odds ratios (ORs) of sleep problems regarding IA status were extracted (where possible) from primary studies. *If these data were not provided*，crude and adjusted ORs with information concerning the confidence interval (CI)，mean, and SD of sleep scores for both groups of normal and internet addicted participants were extracted. Additionally，some studies reported Pearson correlation coefficients between these variables，which were also extracted.

示例 5 - 14　缺失值处理方法——联系作者获取

If data cannot be extracted from the paper or calculated from available information，*we contacted the authors* via email.

此外，对于包含多个时间点测量值的研究，需要说明提取的是哪个时间点的数据，且注意保持一致。如示例 5 - 15 所示，本综述中，由于不同的研究在不同的时间点对研究结果进行了评估，为保持清晰和一致性，该综述着重提取了离干预结束最近的一个时间点的数据。

示例 5 - 15　数据提取说明及缺失值处理方法

Variabilities in the timing and frequencies of outcome measures were anticipated among different studies. For clarity and consistency, we focused on study outcomes that were collected closest to the end of the intervention. Data were extracted *from the graphs* if not reported in the text.

在撰写这一部分时候，需要说明数据提取由几个人完成，是否是独立完成。如果出现不一致的地方，如何处理。如示例 5 - 16 所示，本综述中，多名作者参与到了数据提取过程中。

示例 5 - 16　数据提取参与人员

Full text review and data extraction. Following initial screening, full text was reviewed for final eligibility by a group of 8 reviewers (AA, BH, JY, LD, LG, LM, PT, RJ). Each article was reviewed independently by two reviewers. If either of the two reviewers rated the article as eligible, the article was included for data extraction.

7. 质量评价

纳入文献的研究设计不同，其所需要使用到的文献评估工具也不同。针对 RCT，可以参考 Cochrane 的 Risk of Bias 2 Tool（RoB 2）。该工具从 5 个领域对某一研究的质量进行评价，包括：Bias arising from the randomization process，Bias due to deviations from intended interventions，Bias due to missing outcome data，Bias in measurement of the outcome，Bias in selection of the reported result。每个领域内包含一系列的"信号"问题，通过回答这些问题对相关风险进行判断。基于以上答案，对各个领域的偏倚进行判定，包括"低""高"及"不清楚"。该工具的具体使用方法，可以参看 Cochrane 网站：https://methods.cochrane.org/bias/resources。

类似地，针对非随机试验，也可采用 Cochrane 的工具进行质量评价：Risk of Bias in Non-Randomized Studies of Interventions

（ROBINS-I）。该工具从 7 个领域对某研究的质量进行评价，包括：confounding，selection bias，Bias in measurement classification of interventions，Bias due to deviations from intended interventions，Bias due to missing data，Bias in measurement of outcomes，Bias in selection of the reported result. 每个领域内包含一系列的"信号"问题，通过回答这些问题对相关风险进行判断。基于以上答案，对各个领域的偏倚进行判定，包括"低""中""中高""高"及"不清楚"。该工具的具体使用方法，可以参看 Cochrane 网站：https://methods.cochrane.org/bias/resources。

针对非实验性研究（横断面研究、队列研究及病例对照）的质量评价，可采用 Ottawa-Newcastle Scale（NOS）或者 Joanna Briggs Institute（JBI）中的工具。NOS 及其修订版可从 3 个领域对各研究质量进行评价，包括：研究对象的选择、可比性、结果测量的准确性。根据研究设计，每个领域总分（使用"star"表示）有所不同。分数越高，表明研究质量越高。针对不同的非实验性研究，JBI 包含不同的工具。例如，对于横断面研究，该工具采用了 8 个问题，对该研究的质量进行评价。每个问题相应的回答包括：是、否、不清楚、不适用。根据对 8 个问题的综合评估，确定是否将该研究纳入最终的文献综述中。该工具的具体使用方法，见相关网站：https://joannabriggs.org/critical-appraisal-tools。

在使用以上研究质量评价工具时，需要注意：①多数情况下，质量评价需要由两名研究人员独立开展，以减少主观偏倚。②质量评价结果可以用来指导数据分析、研究结果的解释。此外，有些系统文献综述，会将"研究质量"作为纳入和排除标准。当然，有些综述会把所有符合标准的研究均纳入分析。不管采用何种方案，只要给出合理的原因和解释即可。

如示例 5-17 所示，本综述采用了不同的工具，对不同类型的研究质量进行了评价。并根据研究的质量，确定是否将该研究纳入综述中：对于干预性和观察性研究，不论其质量如何，均将其纳入；对于病历报告，仅纳入了高质量研究。

示例 5 - 17　将研究质量作为纳入标准

Quality assessments were conducted by two independent reviewers (Y. M. B. and D. S.) using modified versions of the Critical Appraisal Skills Programme quality assessment tool for randomized controlled trials (52) and cohort studies (53) and the Joanna Briggs Institute Checklist for case reports. (54) High quality was stated as at least 14 out of 17 points for interventional studies, at least 11 out of 14 points for observational studies, and at least 7 out of 8 points for case reports. These cut-points were established by the review team considering the most relevant items of the checklists. All interventional and observational studies were included irrespective of quality score. Only high-quality case reports were included.

　　如示例 5 - 18 所示，本综述对所有质性研究进行了回顾。但是，并未针对研究质量设置纳入或排除标准。该综述纳入了所有符合条件的文献（不管质量如何）。

示例 15 - 18　纳入所有研究（不论其质量如何）

Eligible studies were appraised for methodological quality using the JBI Critical Appraisal Checklist for Qualitative Research. (40) The checklist consists of 10 criteria concerning the methodology, methods and findings of qualitative studies.

Three members of the review team participated in this step,
and each paper was appraised independently by two of them.
Discrepancies that arose between the reviewers were resolved
through discussion. No studies were excluded based on
methodological quality.

如示例 5-19 所示,本综述纳入了所有符合条件的文献(不管质量如何),但是,在数据提取和分析阶段,对研究质量进行了限定:仅对质量较好的研究进行了数据提取和分析。

示例 5-19　数据提取和分析阶段考虑研究质量

The critical appraisal of original papers was conducted
independently by two reviewers (JK and MW) based on
evaluation criteria adapted from Fortin et al. [12], used to
assess methodological quality (Supplementary data,
Supplement 2). Each article was scored out of 30, based on
criteria on originality, population studied, definition and
measurement of multimorbidity and HrQoL, and limitations
of the study. Risk of bias was assessed using an adapted
version of the Newcastle-Ottawa Scale (NOS) [21]
(Supplementary data, Supplement3) suitable for observational
studies, with good reliability and face validity [22]. Studies
with scores of at least 15 out of 30 using the Fortin checklist,
and 4 out of 9 stars using the NOS were eligible for data
extraction and synthesis.

如示例 5 - 20 所示,本综述纳入了所有符合条件的文献(不管质量如何),但是,在数据分析阶段,考虑了研究质量。该综述采用了敏感性分析,检验低质量研究对研究结果稳定性的影响。

示例 5 - 20 数据分析阶段考虑研究质量

The quantitative meta-analyses were conducted using the Review Manager software (RevMan 5. 3). The first included all studies and a within-groups calculation. The second involved studies with follow-up measures. They were sub-grouped and the effect size was calculated considering any long-lasting effects for DMT with this client population. The third calculation included only studies with RCT designs and between-group scores. Finally, studies with low risk of bias were included in the last calculation that involved a sensitivity analysis.

在撰写质量评价这一部分时,可以通过以下几个方面介绍:介绍不同类型的研究所使用到的质量评价工具;对各个评价工具的主要评估内容及评分标准进行介绍,同时说明所得分数代表的含义;说明质量评价由几个人开展,遇到意见不一致时,是如何处理的。

8. 数据分析方法

在撰写数据分析方法这一部分时,注意内容的完整性和相关性。一般多包含以下几个方面:①数据分析软件(标明版本、软件公司及国家、地区);②如果是 meta-analysis,需要给出具体的数据量化整合方法,例如:以森林图的形式展示各研究及汇总后(pooled)的结果;

③说明缺失值的处理方法(例如,根据已有数据计算而来、通过联系作者获得等);④说明是否进行亚组分析(以及进行此分析的依据)、敏感性分析以及发表偏倚分析。此外,对于无法进行量化的结果,可采用质性方式进行总结,也需对此进行说明。以下将对几个案例着重进行介绍。如示例 5 - 21 所示,该综述根据干预类型进行了亚组分析。如示例 5 - 22 所示,该综述未进行亚组分析,并说明了相应的原因。如示例 5 - 23 所示,该综述对发表偏倚进行了评估,并进行了敏感性分析。

示例 5 - 21　亚组分析

Subgroup analyses were conducted based on the type of intervention: total sleep deprivation (TSD) where participants were completely deprived of any sleep or partial sleep restriction (PSR) where participants' sleep was reduced relative to a basal amount. Additional subgroup analysis was conducted based on sex and the methods of assessment (wherever applicable).

示例 5 - 22　无亚组分析及其原因

For this paper, we also considered the type of subgroup analysis performed in the Meekums et al. (2015) study based on age, but chose not to pursue this mainly due to the fact that only one study survived scrutiny that did not involve adults; this one study was also assessed as having high risk of bias. Subgroup analysis for the type of intervention was not performed either because there were no obvious differences between DMT practices used in the reviewed studies. Finally, although there were differences in the severity of depression at the start of the study，subgroup analysis on the level of depression was not performed because of the limited number of studies；differences were discussed in the narrative meta-synthesis.

示例 5 - 23　发表偏倚及敏感性分析

Publication bias or reporting bias was assessed using the funnel plot alongside the Begg's Test and Eggers' Test. Sensitivity analysis was examined by the Jackknife Method. In this method，which is also known as the 'one out method'，the quality and consistency of the results were evaluated by removing each study individually.

第 5 节　结果和讨论

对于系统文献综述，撰写研究结果和讨论时的技巧与其他类型的论文类似。具体可参考**第 2 章第 4 节和第 5 节**，这里仅对需要额外注意的地方进行说明。

与原创性研究有所不同，在撰写综述的结果时，要注意对各个研究结果的整合，尤其是当无法进行 meta-analysis 时。这里需要达到一个平衡：一方面要保证汇报的全面性；另一方面，又不可对所纳入文献的全部结果进行逐条汇报，否则读者很难抓住论文的重点。

在撰写结果时，可采取以下顺序撰写。首先，介绍文献检索结果,需汇报从初步检索到最终纳入分析的文献数量。结合 PRISMA 流程图进行介绍,无须重复流程图里介绍的全部内容,仅展示核心内容。**其次**,介绍纳入文献的基本特点,一般需要对各个研究总的样本量进行汇总。其余的内容,可根据表格中所展示的信息,进行分类汇总。**再次**,对质量评价结果进行汇报(这个部分,也可以放在前面介绍,注意逻辑性、层次性和流畅性)。**最后**,介绍主要研究结果。如果采用了 meta-analysis,一般多采用森林图的形式展示;如果进行了敏感性分析、亚组分析或评估了发表偏倚,需提供相关结果。

下面以既往发表的一篇文献为例。本研究主要目的是"The aim of this systematic review is to summarize the effect of Mediterranean diet on serum metabolic indices and anthropometric measures among NAFLD patients",如示例 5 - 24 所示,研究结果包含了以下几个方面(这里仅展示了小标题及每个段落的统领句):文献检索结果,各研究的特点(作者先对各研究的基本特点进行了总结,并在同一段落介绍了各个研究的质量;紧接着,在此小标题下,又通过采用次级标题的形式,对主要结果进行汇报)。

示例 5 - 24 研究结果展示形式

3.1 Database search

The literature search yielded 1142 studies, after removing duplicates (Fig. 1).

3.2 Study characteristics

The included trials were conducted between 2008[29] and 2018[30, 31]... The quality of the study was measured by using the Jadad score.

3.2.1 Anthropometric variables

3.2.2 Lipid profile variables...

与原创性研究论文类似,系统文献综述的讨论部分也可以按照以下逻辑书写:概括段;针对主要研究结果分段进行讨论;说明研究的优势或特色(strengths)及局限性(limitations);研究的启示(对于未来的科研及临床实践有何指导意义);结论。各个段落的具体撰写要点,参见**第 2 章**相关内容,这里仅举例进行说明。同样,以上述论文为例,本研究的主要目的是"The aim of this systematic review is to summarize the effect of Mediterranean diet on serum metabolic indices and anthropometric measures among NAFLD patients"。

讨论包含了以下几个方面:总结概述(示例 5 - 25,这里仅展示了这个段落的核心内容),说明本综述的创新性、主要内容及主要研究发现;此外,还针对主要结果展开了相应的讨论;同时,给出了本综述特色和局限性(示例 5 - 26 和示例 5 - 27);小结。

示例 5 - 25　讨论的总结概述段

To the best of our knowledge, no systematic review has been published to assess the effects of MD on serum metabolic profile and anthropometric measures among NAFLD patients. Therefore, we gathered all the interventional studies, which assessed the effectiveness of MD on NAFLD. The present study included 10 randomized controlled trials, which involved a total of 856 adults with NAFLD. In the present systematic review, it was found that...

示例 5 - 26　综述的特色

This systematic review has **some strength**; there is no previous systematic review that assessed the effect of a Medi-

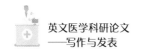

terranean diet on metabolic parameters in patients with non-alcoholic fatty liver disease. Included RCTs were performed in different countries; therefore, differences in lifestyle were considered. There was no limitation for time and language in our systematic review.

示例 5 - 27　综述的局限性举例 1

There are **some limitations** to this study that should be taken into account. First, *significant heterogeneity* was present between the included studies. Heterogeneity may be explained by different and mostly small sample size, different methods for assessment of NAFLD severity, duration of intervention and different ways to encounter control group. Second, there was variability in the control diets; therefore, we could not perform a meta-analysis to quantify the result. The limited number of included studies was also another limitation. Fourth, the effect of sex was not investigated in this review because *none of the studies* reported its result separately on female and male.

　　值得注意的是,系统文献综述的局限性这一部分与原始文献有所不同。它不仅需要包含综述层面的局限性,还要考虑所纳入的各个研究所具有的局限性(这也与 PRISMA checklist 要求的内容一致)。如示例 5 - 27 所示,本综述在综述层面的局限性(例如,所纳入各个研究之间的显著异质性及样本量偏小)和各研究本身存在的局限性(例如,未根据性别进行分析)。当然,也有作者着重介绍综述中所纳入各个研究本身存在的局限性,如示例 5 - 28 所示:研究多采用了横断面研究设计;研究对象多是学生和亚裔,人群代表性不强;主观测量存在局限性等。

示例 5 - 28   综述的局限性举例 2

There are **some limitations** in this meta-analysis. **First**, as mentioned earlier, 22 of 23 analyzed studies were cross-sectional studies, which cannot provide evidence in causality. **Second**, the majority of the participants were students and Asians, which restricts the present review's generalizability. **Third**, all the analyzed studies used self-reports in assessing IA or sleep. Therefore, well-known biases such as social desirability and memory recall bias cannot be excluded. **Finally**, this review cannot draw definitive conclusions concerning the effect of Internet addiction on circadian rhythm and the stability of sleep-wake schedules due to the lack of empirical evidence.

此外,撰写研究的启示一般多从两个方面开展:今后的科学研究以及临床实践(或者卫生政策)。根据期刊要求不同,有些要求作者在讨论中给出启示之后,还会要求使用"**要点**"的形式,说明本研究的启示。如示例 5 - 29 所示,作者从 3 个方面提出了本综述对临床实践的启示。如示例 5 - 30 所示,作者从 4 个方面提出了本综述对未来研究的启示。

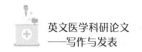

示例 5 - 29　综述对未来临床实践的启示要点

Practice points

1. Internet addiction may result in sleep problems, including lowered sleep quality and reduced sleep duration.

2. Current evidence demonstrates that the association between internet addiction and sleep disturbances exists across different countries, cultures, and ethnicities.

3. Using robust standardized psychometric measures (rather than self-designed measures) in assessing internet addiction and sleep quality is recommended. Standardized measures can ensure the validity and stability in assessing internet addiction and sleep.

示例 5 - 30　综述对未来研究的启示要点

Research agenda

1. Using longitudinal designs and/or randomized controlled trials to assess the causality between internet addiction and sleep can provide healthcare providers direction in treating people with internet addiction problems or those with sleep problems.

2. Most of the studies included in the present meta-analysis comprised students and Asians, Therefore, studies on large samples of Caucasians and those in other age groups are needed to examine whether the association between internet addiction and sleep is consistent across ethnicities and age groups.

3. Studies on reducing or preventing internet addiction are needed to investigate whether the reduced internet addiction can help improve sleep.

4. Impacts of different types of internet addiction are needed to understand which types of internet addiction contribute most to the sleep problems.

第 6 节　其他要点

对于符合纳入和排除标准的论文,可以把他们放在文献整理软件(如,Endnote 或 Refworks)中进行归档,也可以打印出来单独存放,以促进后期数据提取。系统文献综述是对既往研究的分析和评论,对于原始文献所汇报内容的提取是完成一个文献综述的核心步骤。拿到一篇文献之后,可以着重阅读以下几个方面,进行有效数据提取。

首先,通过阅读研究背景,找到研究问题或目的。**其次,**反复阅读研究的方法学,直到能够读懂作者在该研究中做了什么。有时候,由于期刊的篇幅有限,有些重要信息可能无法完全展示在论文里。此时,可以记录下自己的推断(并标记好是自己通过上下文推断出来的)。在方法学中,着重寻找以下信息:研究设计、样本量、纳入和排除标准、研究对象的招募场所、招募和筛查方法、数据收集的具体方法(随访、失访等信息)、主要变量及测量方法等。**再者,**阅读研究结果。在阅读结果时,要重新熟悉本研究的目的,以查看作者是否回答了他们最初提出的研究问题或假设。在回答主要研究问题的过程中,是否提出并回答了其他问题。**然后,**阅读讨论部分。在这一部分,主要考虑研究的优势和局限性,特别注意有哪些其他研究问题还未得到解决。**最后**，还需要关注纳入论文的参考文献列表，进而识别出需要进一步去查阅的论文（包括原创性研究和综述）。

通过采用"data matrix"（数据矩阵）的方式，对所提取的信息进行整理。对文献进行回顾时，常常需要处理太多的细节和信息，如果不对其进行标准化提取和整理，很容易遗漏重要信息且让人觉得数据太杂乱而手足无措。构建数据矩阵如同盖房子，每个单元格里的数据就像一块砖头，通过把每个单元格按照逻辑顺序填满，可以高效地完成数据提取。

构建数据矩阵是撰写综述的基础，可以将其划分为三个主要过程：①有序组织纳入的各个研究：一般多按照发表年限进行组织、排序；②确定提取主题（topic），即确定"表头"，例如：国家、研究目的、研究设计、研究方法等；③阅读每一篇文献，按照表头提取信息。如果有特别需要说明的地方，做好相应的记录。

在构建矩阵时，建议尽可能多地涵盖所要提取的内容。这样的话，有利于避免后期返工。另外，不是每一篇论文都会提供矩阵中拟提取的信息。此时，可以把该研究相对应的那个单元格空在那里。等到完成所有纳入文献的数据提取后，如果大部分论文针对某个内容均未进行汇报，那么在呈现最后的表格时，可以不包含此部分。但是，几乎对于所有的文献综述，都需要提取以下内容：作者、年份、国家。剩余的内容多要依赖于综述的目的以及你对该领域的熟悉程度。在确定剩余要提取的内容时，可以参考以下过程。①阅读纳入的文献：第一遍，按照时间顺序阅读各个文献，这有利于你了解相关研究问题随着时间的变化趋势。第二遍，重点阅读需要提取的部分。②列出重要内容：阅读原始文档时，列出最重要的内容，包括研究方法和特定的内容。例如，如果前面几个研究采用了观察性研究设计，而后来的研究使用了实验性研究设计，那么方法学中的"研究设计"就是一个你需要提取的主题。但是，如果所有的研究都采用了同样的研究设计，呈现结果时，就没有必要单独给出一列展示"研究设计",这样可以减少表格篇幅。③阅读完所有论文以后,请从以下两个方面考虑,进而选择最重要和最相关的主题:该领域的主要内容及文献综述的目的。例如,假设你的文献综述的主要内容是调查治疗失眠的非药物疗法及其效果,那么就需要预留出一栏以提取各种非药物疗法的具体内容。

当然,以下情况也经常发生。在完成了前几个研究的数据提取之后,可能需要添加一些重要的主题(栏目)。添加这些主题后,需要重新查看之前已经完成了数据提取的文献,并对数据矩阵(或表格)进行相应的补充。数据提取是一个反复的过程(iterative process),几乎没有人能够读一遍论文就把所有需要包含的数据提取完。对于所要提取数据的全面性,没有一个一成不变的规则,唯一的指南是:你需要对相关领域的文献足够了解(own the literature),而采用数据矩阵是一个很好的方法。

最后,在开展系统文献综述之前,需要格外注意以下几点(表5-2)。只有明确了开展文献综述过程中的重要任务,并及时规避常见错误,才能够有的放矢,完成一个完整、严谨的系统综述。

表5-2 开展系统文献综述的重要任务及常见错误

重要任务	常见错误
明确研究问题	研究问题过于宽泛(无法回答)
确定开展此综述的必要性(明确是否已有类似综述?)	未及时发现前期已经发表过的类似综述,导致本综述简单地重复既往工作
撰写并注册综述方案(protocol)	没能实现综述的"透明性"
熟悉 PRISMA 指南	未能明确给出纳入和排除标准
详细、完整地提取研究信息	遗漏研究重要信息或数据
数据分析(文字总结或 meta-analysis)	没能识别并汇报纳入研究间存在的异质性
对纳入文献进行质量评价	没能识别并汇报纳入研究存在的偏倚
明确给出综述的主要发现	结论过大,超出了综述所涵盖的范围

第 **6** 章　医学论文的撰写格式

　　撰写论文是一项艰巨的任务。能把论文写完就是一件值得庆祝的事情。然而,如果能在论文撰写过程中注意到一些细节,往往会为论文增色不少。在投稿指南中,杂志往往会对稿件的撰写细节及参考文献格式提出一些要求,要求作者遵循一定的格式。对于医学类期刊而言,常常要求作者在书写论文时采用 APA 格式(American Psychological Association style)或 AMA 格式(American Medical Association style)。关于这两种书写格式,美国心理学会出版的 *Publication Manual of the American Psychological Association* (*7ᵗʰ edition*)及美国医学会出版的 *American Medical Association Manual of Style：A Guide to Authors and Editors* (*11ᵗʰ edition*)有详细的描述,建议读者自备,作为工具书,可随时查询。与 APA 格式相比,AMA 格式相对比较简单。在 AMA 格式中,每篇参考文献都对应着唯一的数字编号,在参考文献列表中每篇文献按在文中出现的先后顺序进行排列,在正文中则是根据出现顺序用数字上标进行引用。鉴于篇幅所限,本章将重点对 APA 格式需要格外注意的地方进行介绍。本章中,我们将主要回答以下两个问题。

- 对于论文格式,APA 有哪些一般要求?
- 对于参考文献,APA 有哪些具体要求?

第1节　APA 格式一般要求

APA 格式是一种被广泛接受的研究型论文撰写格式,起源于 1929 年,由具有学术权威性的美国心理学会(American Psychological Association,APA)发布。该格式主要用于心理学、护理学、教育学、社会科学领域的论文写作。2019 年 10 月,美国心理学会发布了第 7 版《APA 发表手册》(*Publication Manual*),取代了 2009 年发布的第 6 版。目前如果投稿的话,期刊一般都要求遵循第 7 版而不是第 6 版的要求。为了让大家尽快熟悉最新的要求,本章节会根据第 7 版手册上面的内容进行介绍,重点介绍与中文写作习惯不一样的地方。鉴于部分读者已有投稿经验且比较了解第 6 版,在涉及第 7 版和第 6 版的不同之处,本章节会做特别提醒。

论文布局相关格式要求(layout)

正文格式:APA 格式的论文最多可包括 5 级标题,3 级标题的居多。1 级标题居中、粗体;2 级标题左对齐、粗体;3 级标题左对齐、粗体、斜体。各级标题均使用 title case 的格式(什么是 title case,详见**第 2 章第 1 节**)。前言段落默认 1 级标题为"Introduction",但是不需要写出这个单词,因此,前言中的段落如需加标题,则从 2 级标题开始。

行间距:一般情况下,全文采用双倍行距(表格可以使用单倍、1.5 倍或双倍行距,根据排版情况而定),左对齐。每个段落的第一行缩进 0.5 英寸,使用 Tab 键或者 Word 程序默认的分段落时自动首行缩进。注意:不要使用空格键空四个格。关于纸张的设置,四边的页边距均为 1 英寸,即 2.54 cm。

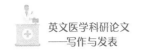
字体字号：全文所使用的字体及字号大小包括 Calibri 11 号，Arial 11 号，Lucida Sans Unicode 10 号，Times New Roman 12 号，Georgia 11 号，不再像第 6 版仅限于 Times New Roman 12 号。

标点符号：①在逗号、句号、分号和冒号后面需要空一格再接后面的内容。例如，使用 it includes：A and B 而非 it includes：A and B。②在三个及以上并列的单词之间使用逗号，并且最后一个单词前应使用 and，在 and 之前应有逗号。例如，使用 height，width，and depth 而非 height，width and depth。③当描述数字时，每三位数用逗号隔开，例如，1,000,000。当表示日期时，如日期具体到天，则在天和年之间加逗号，例如，On January 14,2021；如果只有年份和月份，则不需要逗号，例如，In January 2021。④用双引号而非斜体来引用语言示例，比如：APA endorses the use of singular pronoun "they"而非 APA endorses the use of the singular pronoun *they*。

时态：在描述既往研究结果、结论及研究方法、实验流程时，使用一般过去时或现在完成时。在描述研究结果时，采用一般过去时。在讨论结果的意义、研究结论、研究局限性及未来研究方向时则采用一般现在时。

语态：APA 格式允许使用主动语态和被动语态，但提倡尽可能使用主动语态，避免过度使用被动语态。如果强调动作的承受者时，可以使用被动语态。

避免拟人化：例如，可以使用 the theory addresses 而非 the theory concludes；因为 theory 可以 address、indicate 或 present，但不能 conclude，只有人（即研究者）才能 conclude。类似地，使用 we investigated 而非 this study investigated。

关于"they"的使用：避免使用 he/she、s/he、(s)he 或 he or she，尤其是在性别不明的情况下，用 they 来代替。例如，Each participant turned in their questionnaire 而非 Each participant turned in his or her questionnaire。

量表赋值：介绍量表的赋值时，选项用斜体表示。例如，Students were asked to rate each instructor as *poor*（1），*fair*（2），*good*（3），*very good*（4），or *excellent*（5）。

连接号的使用：表示数值范围时，两个数字间用连接号（En dash-），而不是连字符（hyphen-）或破折号（Em dash—）相连。在 Word 中，先输入数字 2013，然后再同时按住 alt 键和字母 X 键，即可得到连接号"–"。例如：正确的表示方法是 items 1–7，而不是 items 1-7 或 items 1—7。当表示两个百分比的范围时，两个数字后均应保留％符号。应该是 60％—80％而非 60—80％。

范围：在介绍范围时，建议给出确切的年龄范围而非广泛的类别。例如，使用 People in the age range of 60 to 70 years old 而非 People over 60 years old.

人群描述：避免使用形容词来标记人群（易造成污名化），尽量使用描述性短语。例如，使用 patients with diabetes 而非 diabetic patients；使用 people living in poverty 而非 the poor。

引文：对于整段的引用，各行均需缩进 0.5 英寸（即 1.27 cm）。如果引用了两段内容，则第二段比第一段又要缩进 0.5 英寸。

图表：图表的编号、标题及标注（note）均为左对齐，图表标题及"note"一词均为斜体。图表的编号与标题各占一行。图表采用三线表，没有竖线。

标题：标题避免使用缩写；避免使用"a study of"或"an experimental investigation of"之类无意义的字眼。标题中，各单词的书写需要使用 title case，具体要求可参看本书**第 2 章第 1 节**。

姓名：APA 格式推荐论文作者的书写格式为名在前，姓在后。例如，Keke Lin。对于有些国家的作者，名与姓之间还可能有中间名，可用首字母缩写表示，例如，Carol J. Smith。

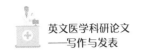

第2节 APA 格式的参考文献格式要求

APA 格式的参考文献格式要求涉及正文中的引文（Citations in Text）和文末的参考文献列表（Reference List）两大部分。下面，将对需要特别注意的地方进行介绍。

1. 正文中引文格式

● APA 格式的引文采用的是 in-text citation 的形式，即：在文中引用资源时，要写明该资源的作者及日期。如为直接引用，还需要标明页码，单页用"p."，多页用"pp."表示。

● 正文中所有引用的材料必须出现在参考文献列表中（质性研究中研究对象的原话等除外）。同理，文末列表中给出的参考文献也必须在正文中引用过。

● 正文中引用的资源来自相同作者（指作者数量及顺序均相同）同一年份的多篇文献时，需要在年份后加 a、b、c 等进行区分。区分的标准为文献标题第一个单词首字母的顺序，在参考文献列表中亦按字母顺序罗列这些文献。例如，(Zhu, 2019a, 2019b)。来自同一作者不同年份的文献时，则按年份由远至近的顺序进行排列。例如，(Zhu, 2019, 2020)；年份不明的放在最前面，例如，(Zhu, n. d. , 2019, 2020)。

● 在正文中引用的资源有两个作者时，如果是在信号短语（signal phrase，例如，according to, as cited by）中标注的话，一般是将这两个作者用"and"连接起来。例如，According to Zhu and Lin (2021)。如果是放在括号中，则用"&"相连。例如，(Zhu & Lin, 2021)。

● 正文引用三个及以上作者，全部用 et al. ，不再像第 6 版规定的那样（第一次引用时，给出全部作者；第二次引用时，才使用 et al.）。例如，正文中正确的引用方式是（Lin，et al.，2017）而非（Lin，Park，Li，Wang & Quinn，2017）。

- 如作者为某个组织且该组织有简称时，第一次出现时需要给出全称，同时标出简称，在之后的引用中直接使用简称。例如，第一次引用时［National Institute of Health（NIH），2019］，之后的引用中直接使用（NIH，2019）。

2. 文末参考文献格式

- 参考文献（References）应放在正文"Conclusion"后，图表及附录前。参考文献需另起一页，按第一作者姓氏的首字母顺序给出，而非按文献在文中出现的顺序给出。若第一作者姓氏首字母相同，则按名的首字母缩写顺序进行排列。
- 同一条参考文献的各行以及各条参考文献之间均为双倍行距。每条参考文献的非首行左侧均需要缩进 0.5 英寸。
- 对于包含多个作者的参考文献，第 7 版规定：如有 2～20 名（含）作者时，需要全部列出，最后一名作者与倒数第二名作者之间用 & 相连。例如，Lin，K.，Zhu，B.，Smith，C.，Wang，L.，Li，M.，Zheng，G.，Quinn，L.，Collins，E.，Ferrans，C.，Park，C.，Park，M.，Liu，Y.，Shi，C.，Meng，J.，Wang，H.，Li，Z.，Hao，Y.，Yue，S.，Sun，Y. & Zhou F.（2021）。如有 21 名及以上作者，则先列出前 19 名作者，之后使用...而不是 &，继而列出最后一名作者。例如，前例中如作者多于 20 名，则参考文献应列为 Lin，K.，Zhu，B.，Smith，C.，Wang，L.，Li，M.，Zheng，G.，Quinn，L.，Collins，E.，Ferrans，C.，Park，C.，Park，M.，Liu，Y.，Shi，C.，Meng，J.，Wang，H.，Li，Z.，Hao，Y.，Yue，S.，Sun，Y.，...Zhou F.（2021）。
- 参考文献列表中期刊的名称需要列全，不可采用缩写。期刊名称使用的大小写及符号应跟原期刊一致。例如，Journal of Midwifery & Women's Health 不可写成 JMWH 或 Journal of Midwifery and Women's Health。此外，期刊名及卷数需使用斜体。

● 与第 6 版不同，第 7 版中，参考文献中无须提供出版社地理位置。

● 参考文献部分 doi 全部采用 URLs 格式，不再像第 6 版可以使用"doi："。例如，使用 http://dx. doi. org/10. 1016/j. diabres. 2017. 03. 013 而非 doi：10. 1016/j. diabres. 2017. 03. 013。

APA 格式对参考文献在文中的引文及文末的列表要求较多。建议使用文献管理软件(例如，Endnote)辅助：生成参考文献列表时选择 APA(第七版)，则会自动生成符合 APA(第七版)要求的引文及参考文献列表，而不需要手动去输入。使用文献管理软件的另外一个优势在于能自动转换参考文献格式，比如从 APA 格式转换成 AMA 格式，这在论文需要改投他刊时比较方便。但是，经过文献管理软件格式化之后的参考文献列表，还会存在细节上的问题。例如，期刊首字母未大写、标题格式错误。因此，有必要进行人工核对。此外，有时候会出现两种格式不兼容、转换格式出错的情况，这时也需要人工核对。因此，有必要熟悉 APA 格式对参考文献的要求。

除了纸质版工具书 *Publication Manual of the American Psychological Association*（*7ᵗʰ edition*），还可以参考网络资源 https：//apastyle. apa. org/。该网站是介绍 APA 格式的官方网站，提供了大量的免费范例和视频，供有兴趣的读者进一步浏览学习。同时，该网站还免费提供质性研究(JARS-Qual)、量性研究(JARS-Quant)和混合研究(JARS-Mixed)的论文书写格式，相关网站如下：https：//apastyle. apa. org/jars。当然，很多杂志在投稿须知中也会提供论文撰写的模板，可以直接把模板下载下来后在模板上进行写作。

APA 格式较其他论文书写格式略显烦琐，对于初学者而言需要使用一段时间才能慢慢适应。但是,本章所述的格式要求基本能够满足初学者的需求。在今后的写作过程中遇到其他格式问题时,再查询纸质工具书或网络资源,慢慢积累经验,则会在使用 APA 格式时越来越得心应手。

第7章 投稿及发表

正如第1章所述,科学研究过程中的另一个重要环节是将研究结果进行"推广与分享"。对于处于科研生涯起步阶段的学生或研究人员来说,可以通过参加国内外学术会议或在科研组会/研讨会中分享自己的研究成果。但将论文发表在同行评议的学术期刊中仍然是一种十分常见且重要的形式。完成了论文撰写之后,下一步就是进行投稿和发表。本章中,我们将通过回答以下问题,简要介绍论文的投稿与发表过程中可采用的技巧及需要避免的误区。

- 如何选择合适的投稿期刊?
- 投稿过程中需要准备哪些上传材料?
- 投稿后,稿件都有哪些状态?
- 论文为何被拒?
- 如何对一篇论文进行修回?
- 论文被接收后,还有哪些工作需要完成?

第1节 选择合适的期刊

有时候,选择目标期刊比写好一篇论文更重要。在声誉差的期刊上发表论文可能会降低研究的可信度,并降低研究结果的影响力。

因此,在投稿前,一定要慎重选择合适的期刊。对于没有太多投稿经验的人来说,为自己的论文选择合适的期刊具有一定的挑战性。结合我们既往的投稿经验,以下因素在选择合适期刊的过程中具有重要的指导意义。

1. 影响因子或分区

一个期刊的影响因子,反映了该期刊在某领域的影响力。任何一篇论文发表出来,都希望能够获得更多的关注。虽然目前的科研评价体系反对"唯影响因子",但不可否认,发表在高影响因子期刊上的论文,其研究内容往往更为深入,研究结论往往具有更高的科学价值,也往往更容易获得同研究领域的关注。因此,影响因子成为很多人选择目标期刊的首要考虑因素。但是,我们认为,在以影响因子为指导方向的时候,需要结合自己的学科或研究领域。以护理为例,该学科最顶级期刊 *Int J Nurs Stud* 的影响因子也仅逾 5 分(2020年),与临床医学或基础医学所涵盖期刊的影响因子完全不具有可比性。但是,其在护理领域的影响力的确是最大的。当然,也有学者反对在选择目标期刊时,以影响因子为导向。在此背景下,有学者提出可以根据"期刊分区"来进行选择。以 Journal Citation Report (JCR)分区为例,此方法将期刊按照其所属学科领域进行分区,包括 Q1 区~Q4 区。Q1 区期刊影响力高于 Q2 区,以此类推。因此,在选择目标期刊时,也可参考期刊分区。

2. 论文与期刊范畴的契合度

我们认为,在选择目标期刊时,论文内容与期刊的范畴及其受众群体(audiences)的契合度,可能比选择期刊的影响因子更加重要。每个期刊所涵盖的范畴或侧重点都有所差异(即使是同一学科),投

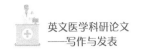

稿指南中的第一部分多会介绍期刊的目的和涵盖范畴。以 *Int J Nurs Stud* 为例(示例 7-1),该期刊的概述中,介绍了期刊的目的、所接受论文的类型、论文可以覆盖的内容以及读者群体。所以,如果你的论文内容上与该期刊范畴不契合,那么不建议投稿。

示例 7-1 *Int J Nurs Stud* 期刊的目的、范畴及受众群体

"The International Journal of Nursing Studies (IJNS) provides a forum for original research and scholarship about health care delivery, organization, management, workforce, policy and research methods relevant to nursing, midwifery and other health related professions."

"The IJNS **aims** to support evidence-informed policy and practice by **publishing research, systematic and other scholarly reviews, critical discussion, and commentary** of the highest standard. The journal particularly welcomes studies that aim to evaluate and understand complex health care interventions and health policies and which employ the most rigorous designs and methods appropriate for the research question of interest. The journal also seeks to advance the quality of research by publishing **methodological papers** introducing or elaborating on analytic techniques, measures, and research methods."

"**Audience**: Nurses, midwives, educators, administrators and researchers in all areas of nursing and caring sciences."

随着临床医学亚专业的细化,与多个亚学科相应的期刊也应运而生,这也是投稿时需要考虑的一点。例如,如果你的论文是与糖尿

病临床治疗或护理相关的,那么就不适合投稿于仅接收基础论文的期刊。当然,如果你的研究是交叉学科研究,则可以同时从两个或多个领域中选择目标期刊(例如,你的研究调查了糖尿病患者中血糖与骨质疏松的关系)。此外,所选择期刊也可以是综合性期刊。此类期刊受众面很广,所接收论文不仅限于某种疾病或某个健康问题。例如, *JAMA* 就是这样一个综合性期刊,接收所有医学相关论文。根据我们的经验,如果你所在的领域中已经有多个可以选择的专业期刊,则尽量先从这些期刊中选择投稿。如果没有合适的,再考虑综合性期刊。

此外,有些期刊不接受综述类论文,或者仅采用"约稿"的形式,或者需要作者在投稿前咨询主编是否对其所要投的综述感兴趣。在选择期刊时,要尤其注意这一点:可以通过阅读投稿指南获取此信息。

3. 熟悉程度和既往经验

对于某期刊的熟悉程度以及既往在该期刊中是否具有投稿经验,也是在选择投稿期刊过程中可以参考的一点。如果你周围的同学或同事(同领域)多数会选择某期刊进行投稿或者某个期刊是你所在领域中公认的投稿期刊,那么可以选择此期刊。当然,还可以咨询你的 co-author(尤其是 senior author)的建议,他们往往在选择期刊方面具有一定的经验。此外,如果你在某期刊上已有过投稿经验,那么你对于该期刊所接收论文的范畴以及投稿指南就会比较熟悉,你也可以选择此期刊投稿。

4. 审稿周期

规范的学术期刊均会给出明确的同行评审过程。例如:同行评审所用的标准、评审人员的选择、同行评审的类型(单盲还是双盲)、同行评审的周期以及编委会如何处理同行评审结果。根据期刊不同,审稿周期有所不同,多数期刊的初审耗时约 1~2 个月,但有些可能需要 3 个月甚至更长。审稿周期的长短也是在选择目标期刊时需要考虑的一点,这对于急需论文发表出来者至关重要。一个期刊的审稿周期,可以从该期刊的官网上查询到,有时候也会在投稿指南上进行介绍。同时,Web of Knowledge 下的 JCR 中,收录了各种 SCI 期刊。你可以选择目标期刊,查询其影响因子,以及该期刊每年发表的论文数,期刊是月刊、双月刊还是旬刊。通过以上数据,你也可以对其审稿周期做出一个预估。

5. 参考文献列表

还有些时候,你完全不知道该选择哪个期刊进行投稿。此时,可以浏览一下你的参考文献列表,大致了解一下你所引用的论文都发表在哪些期刊中,这可能为你提供一定的思路。

6. 其他因素

虽然不是主要影响因素,但是审稿费和版面费也是在选择期刊时需要考虑的因素。多数期刊无须缴纳审稿费和发表费。但是,有些期刊需缴纳审稿费,例如 Mary Ann Liebert 出版商旗下的期刊会收取 49 美元的审稿费。此外,大多数期刊对于彩色图片会收取一定的版面费,这些信息均会在投稿指南中有所介绍。在投稿前,需要仔细阅读投稿指南,进一步确定。

除了以上因素会影响目标期刊的选择,在选择期刊过程中,还需注意避免以下常见行为。

首先,避免以影响因子为风向标。有些作者在投稿时,唯影响因子论,而不考虑自己的论文与期刊涵盖范畴的契合度,这很容易被拒稿。如果在同等有影响力的期刊中进行选择,建议选择与你的论文内容更加一致的期刊。如果一个期刊影响力大于另一期刊,但是影响力小的期刊却与你的论文更加匹配。此时,如果选择影响力小的期刊,那么在编辑处就被拒稿的可能性就较小。相反,如果想要冒险,选择与你的论文匹配度不是很高但是影响因子较高的期刊,则在编辑处被拒稿的可能性就较大。当然,如果你确信你的论文十分具有竞争力,也不妨一试。

其次,避免过度自信。有些作者在投稿时,过度自信,认为自己的论文可以投在影响因子很高的期刊上,但是其研究的特色、创新性和重要性并没有达到其所选期刊的要求。此时,如果你贸然选择该期刊,在主编阶段就被拒稿的可能性就非常大。这不仅会浪费你的时间(因为你在投稿前,需要根据该期刊的投稿指南对论文进行相应的修改),也浪费了编辑的时间。更加重要的是,被拒稿会给你带来很大的心理压力和负担,这种压力甚至会影响你正常的学习和工作。这一点对于初次投稿的人而言十分重要。

再者,避免选择掠夺性期刊(predatory journal)、**假刊或者水刊。**掠夺性期刊是以谋利为目的的期刊,需要作者缴纳高昂的发表费但并不向其提供预期的专业服务(例如,同行评审、编辑、索引等)。为了吸引作者,此类期刊多数会承诺快速发表,接收并发表所有来稿;而且,通常会在论文被接收发表后才告知作者需要缴纳版面费。它们还常常故意使用与知名期刊相似的名称,误导投稿者(尤其是没有投稿经验者)。此外,还有一些假期刊,例如:没有撤稿政策、没有明确说明期刊范围和同行评议过程、通过电子邮件投稿等。需格外注意此类期刊,对其进行甄别。国际医学期刊编辑委员会(International Committee of Medical Journal Editors, ICMJE)建议:在选择期刊时,作者有责任评估所选期刊的历史、规范性和学术声誉。目前,还存在水刊一说。此类期刊多数是OA(open access)期

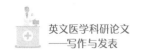

刊,需要缴纳发表费。其发表起来相对简单,也被 SCI 收录,但是其同行评议并不是特别规范,有些高校还针对此类期刊制定了"黑名单"。在投稿前,需要熟悉你所在单位是否对此有所规定。如果实在不清楚,则可以咨询同事或者团队的其他作者。

处于科研生涯初期的学者,如果收到了邮件邀请投稿,多数情况是虚假邮件。邮件内容里多包含如下内容:存在语法错误,过多地使用感叹号、承诺快速审稿及发表、期刊目的及范畴与你的研究领域无关、出版商或会议举办商你没有听说过、期刊名称与已有规范期刊非常相似、编辑或相关工作人员未提供相应的头衔、未提供该期刊的影响因子或用语含糊不清、该期刊没有 ISSN、所发表论文没有 doi号、要求先交版面费或承诺免除版面费。

为了避免误入掠夺性期刊的雷区,在选择期刊时,需要考虑期刊的质量(不仅仅是影响因子)。衡量期刊质量的关键指标是期刊中所发表论文的科学严谨性。在选择目标期刊时,可以回顾一下过去几年该期刊所发表论文的研究设计、具体方法等,进而为你进行评估提供参考。严谨的期刊对于论文的格式、图表、审稿过程等都有明确规定。可帮助评价期刊质量的另一个指标是该期刊是否要求论文按照公认的指南进行报告,例如:CONSORT, PRISMA, STROBE 等;针对临床试验性研究,是否预先进行注册。数据共享政策的透明度也是评估期刊严谨性时可以考虑的一个因素。数据共享对于确保科学研究的透明度和可复制性,以及建立公众信任至关重要。期刊编委的信息也可为评估期刊质量提供一定的参考。编委会成员应是该期刊所属领域内公认的专家,并隶属于正规单位。同时,较严谨的期刊还会发表该期刊主编或编委所撰写的社论(editorial),鼓励针对某特定主题(specific issue)来稿,或为作者与读者介绍本刊在政策上的更新。如果该期刊网站或投稿指南中,未提供编辑联系信息,在选择该刊时,则需要慎重。

第2节　根据投稿指南准备投稿所需清单

　　每一个期刊都会有详细、明确的投稿指南（author guidelines）。该指南中，多数会说明投稿时需要提供的文件清单。所以，在投稿前（甚至是在撰写论文前），一定要仔细阅读目标期刊的投稿指南。多数情况下，需要提供以下文件清单，包括：Cover letter, Title page, Main text, Figure legends, Figures, Tables, Supplements, Conflict of interest form。

1. 如何撰写 Cover letter

　　多数情况下，在投稿阶段，需要提供 Cover letter（个别期刊可能不要求）。虽然各期刊针对 Cover letter 中需要包含的信息在要求上有所不同，但是撰写需要遵循信件的形式。内容上要言简意赅，注意控制字数，一般不超过一页（单倍或 1.2 倍行距）。一般情况下，需要包含以下几个成分：①信件的收信人（Editor-in-Chief or Editor）。②信件的开头：介绍所提交稿件的类型（例如，original paper 或 systematic review）及标题。③信件的主体：对你的研究进行简要介绍，包括研究的大体内容及研究意义。④本研究对该期刊的贡献：说明为什么你的论文适合投在该期刊上。⑤常规性段落：说明没有一稿多投、所有作者都同意投稿等情况，并表示感谢。根据期刊不同，有些要求将作者分工及是否存在利益冲突放在 Title page，有些则要求其放在 Cover letter。此外，越来越多的杂志要求投稿者在 Cover letter 中说明：所投稿件是否与既往已发表论文使用了同一数据（集）。如果是，则要说明此稿件与既往论文有何联系和差别。⑥署名（即写信人，第一作者或通讯作者）。署名时，除了给出作者姓

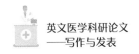
名、学位、头衔,还有给出单位、地址和邮箱。下面的案例中,将分享我们既往投稿中使用的 Cover letter。

Dear Dr. /Prof. . . . ,

We would like to submit an **original paper** entitled "..." in the *Annals of the New York Academy of Sciences*.

Pregnant women frequently experience various sleep disturbances such as altered sleep architecture, short sleep duration, and obstructive sleep apnea... Nonetheless, few studies have examined the relationships between objective sleep and inflammatory biomarkers in pregnant women. Thus, we evaluated the...

We believe that this manuscript is appropriate for publication in the *Annals of the New York Academy of Sciences*. **This study will** enhance our knowledge about the underlying pathways linking sleep and metabolic health. **Findings from this study will** provide invaluable information for a **broad range of readers** including healthcare providers (e. g. , obstetricians, diabetologists, sleep physicians, and nurses) as well as clinically oriented researchers.

The manuscript described here has not been published previously, and is not under consideration for publication elsewhere, in whole or in part. All authors have approved the manuscript.

On behalf of the co-authors, I greatly appreciate your time to review our manuscript.

Sincerely,

Name，title
Institution
Address
Email

2. 撰写 Title page 需要注意什么

根据期刊不同,有些要求作者单独提供 Title page,有些要求作为正文的第一页提供。Title page 的撰写相对比较简单,一般不超过一页。因为各期刊多会对 Title page 中需要提供的信息给出详细的说明,所以按照其要求进行准备,便不会出现问题。这里需要注意以下几点。

(1) 作者及作者顺序:对于采用双盲审稿的期刊,一般要求在提交的稿件正文中隐去作者信息,而把作者信息放在 Title page 中。在投稿阶段,分别提交 Title page 和稿件正文。作者及作者顺序多在开始撰写论文之前就应参考 ICMJE 中的原则确定好(尤其是第一作者、通讯作者和 senior author)。此外,在投稿前,各位作者必须已经认可该顺序,一则因为作者顺序在投稿后一般不能轻易更改,如需更改,需要给编辑部提交更改理由;二则因为 SCI 论文发表涉及各位作者利益,事先认可也是为了避免日后纠纷。在 Title page 中,按照实际情况给出作者顺序。如果存在共同第一或共同通讯的情况,需要进行标注并说明。例如,在共同贡献的名字上使用 # 上标进行标注,同时给出注释:# The authors contributed equally to the preparation of this manuscript and should be considered as joint first authors。

(2) 作者贡献(author contribution):有些期刊要求在 Title page 中,说明每名作者对该论文的贡献。关于作者贡献的撰写格式,可以参考以上对于"作者"标准的规定;还可以参考 CRediT 格式进行撰写,此格式的提出是体现了从 authorship 转变为 contribution-ship,涵盖了研究开展过程中各个阶段的工作及每个作者的贡献,例如:构思、实施、论文撰写、获取基金等。关于 CRediT 的详细介绍,请见相关网站:https://www.elsevier.com/authors/journal-authors/

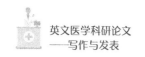
policies-and-ethics/credit-author-statement。常见的两种形式如示例 7 - 2 和示例 7 - 3 所示：第一个示例（示例 7 - 2）是根据传统 ICMJE 对于"作者"定义所撰写的；第二个示例（示例 7 - 3）是按照 CRediT 的形式所撰写的。

示例 7 - 2　作者贡献举例 1

Author contributions

B. Z. contributed to the conception of work, acquisition of data, analysis, and interpretation of data, and participated in drafting the manuscript. B. I. B. contributed to the conception and design of the study, analysis, and interpretation of data, and participated in drafting and revising the manuscript. B. I. B. and B. Z. accept responsibility for the integrity of the data analyzed. U. G. B. , D. W. C. , K. L. , A. S. , and M. C. K. contributed analysis and interpretation of data, and participated in revising the manuscript. All authors approved the final version of the submitted manuscript.

示例 7 - 3　作者贡献举例 2

Author Statement

BZ: Conceptualization; Data curation; Formal analysis; Funding acquisition; Original draft.

YY: Conceptualization; Methodology; Review & editing.

CS: Data curation; Formal analysis; Review & editing.

JC: Data curation; Validation; Review & editing.

CP: Formal analysis; Methodology; Review & editing.

XC: Conceptualization; Methodology; Supervision;

Review & editing.

　　IBB：Conceptualization；Methodology；Supervision；Review & editing.

　　（3）作者名字书写格式：先写名，后写姓（例如：朱冰倩，Bingqian Zhu）；提供相应的学历及头衔（例如：学历，PhD 或 MS；头衔，MD 或 RN）。

　　（4）单位：给出单位名称，院系，城市，国家，邮编。例如：School of Nursing，Shanghai Jiao Tong University，Shanghai，China，200025。

　　（5）利益冲突声明（conflict of interest）：如果没有利益冲突，可以采用期刊推荐的撰写格式，例如：The authors declare no conflict of interest。如果存在利益冲突，则需要进行说明：谁在哪方面存在利益冲突。例如，既往的一篇系统文献综述中，我们调查了睡眠剥夺对于代谢指标的影响，其中一名作者接受了公司的讲课费，其在文中进行了利益声明。如示例 7 - 4 所示：

示例 7 - 4　利益冲突声明

Conflicts of interest

　　SR receives grant support from Merck Sharp and Dohme, and speaker honoraria from Sanofi, Novo Nordisk, and Medtronic.

　　对潜在的利益冲突进行声明，是科学研究的一个重要但常被忽略的环节。根据 ICMJE：“*The potential for conflict of interest and bias exists when professional judgment concerning a primary interest（e. g. , patients' welfare or the validity of research）may be influenced by a secondary interest（e. g. , financial gain）. Although the presence of a relationship or activity does not always indicate a problematic influence on a paper's content，perceptions of conflict may erode trust in science as much as actual conflicts of interest. An author's complete disclosure demonstrates a commitment to transparency and helps to maintain trust in the scientific process.*"

最常见的利益冲突是"经济性"利益冲突，包括：受雇于某单位、咨询费、讲课费、专利费等。此类利益冲突易于识别，也最容易影响期刊、作者及科学的可信性。此外，还需要尽量避免与营利性或非营利性资助者签订协议，此类协议有可能会影响作者开展研究、分析数据及报告结果等科研活动。故意遗漏潜在的利益冲突，也属于科研不当行为。因此，每位作者均需要报告自己是否存在利益冲突，这也是科研诚信中值得格外注意的地方。多数期刊要求投稿时上传"Conflict of interest form"，常采用的是 ICMJE 所推荐的，相关网站如下：http://icmje. org/conflicts-of-interest/。

（6）致谢（acknowledgement）：根据期刊不同，致谢可以放在 Title page，也可以放在论文末尾、参考文献之前（单独一页）。致谢的对象可以包括：研究对象，为本研究的开展提供了帮助但是达不到"作者"标准的人（例如，帮忙修改语法、对论文提供反馈意见），如示例 7-5 所示。此外，有些期刊要求将课题基金或研究经费来源置于致谢中。经费来源的撰写格式，根据期刊有所不同，在投稿时需关注期刊的投稿指南，如示例 7-6 所示。

示例 7-5　致谢"人"

The authors thank Dr. Alicia K. Matthews, Professor at UIC College of Nursing (Department of Health Systems Science), for the constructive feedback.

示例 7 - 6　致谢"人"和"基金"

The authors thank Mr Luis Antônio Potenza, Mr Pedro Sérgio Simões and Mr Paulo Celso Franco for technical assistance, and Cristiane de Paula Teixeira for the estradiol serum assay. This research was supported by public funding from São Paulo Research Foundation (FAPESP - grant numbers 2012/19428 - 8; 2012/22666 - 8), National Council for Scientific and Technological Development (CNPq) and by Coordination of Improvement of Higher Level Personnel (CAPES), Brazil.

　　注：针对作者贡献、利益声明、致谢、课题基金这几个方面的信息，根据期刊不同，这一部分可以放在 Title page 中或放在文末、参考文献之前。

3. Main text 中所提供的信息需要注意什么

　　个别期刊的审稿过程采用双盲，此时，所提交的正文中不能涉及泄露作者身份的任何信息，包括获得伦理审查的机构及自引论文信息。在继往投稿过程中，我们常采用如下方法：在介绍伦理审查时，未给出详细的单位名称；在引用自己既往发表过的论文时，使用"blinded for peer review"这一写法（在论文被接收后，可以提供该引文相关的全部信息），如图 7 - 1 所示。

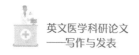
Ethical considerations

The study was approved by the Institutional Review Board of a public university (*Blinded for Peer Review*). All participants provided written informed consent.

The sample size for the parent study was determined a priori by power simulation. In this report, data from 56 participants were analyzed. Detailed inclusion/exclusion criteria and participant recruitment were described elsewhere (*Blinded for Peer Review*).

图 7‑1　Main Text 需要注意的信息

4. 准备 Figures(图)和 Tables(表)时,需要注意什么

根据期刊要求不同,图表在文中的位置有所不同。多数情况下,Figures 多不与正文放在同一个 Word 文档中,而是在投稿过程中单独上传,其格式多为 TIFF、JPG 等。当然,有的期刊允许将 Figures 与正文放在同一个 Word 文档中。在准备 Figures 时,还需要提供 Figure legends 并置于正文的参考文献之后、Tables 之前。相比而言,Tables 可与正文放在同一个 Word 文档中,并置于文中首次提及的地方或文末。如果将图表置于文末,则每个图表均需要从新的一页开始。此外,一般情况下,期刊对于图表总数均有限制。因此,在图表的数量上可能需要有所取舍,能文字说清楚的,则无须图表。具体要求,可参考目标期刊的投稿指南。

5. Supplement 是什么

用于辅助所提交论文的图表、清单等,可以作为 Supplement 上传。个别期刊对于所提供图表的总数有限制,如果论文中包含的图表太多,而无法全部放在正文中,则可以把最重要的放在正文,把剩余的、相对来说没那么重要但又不可缺少的图表放在附录中上传。此外,有些期刊还要求提供论文汇报时所遵循的清单(例如,

PRISMA checklist），此时可以把其作为附录上传。

6. 如何选择审稿人

有些期刊要求投稿时推荐审稿人，这可以帮助编辑找到合适的审稿人。当然，编辑并不一定会将你的论文发给你所推荐的专家进行审稿。所推荐的审稿人需要对你提交稿件所属领域比较熟悉，但不能是熟人（例如，单位同事、知道你此次投稿的专家或以前一起投过稿的专家），这有可能造成利益冲突。在选择审稿专家时，可以采用以下三种方法：①根据你对本领域的了解，选择相关专家。例如，在阅读文献时，你会读到许多与你的研究相关的论文，这些论文的作者可以作为潜在的审稿人。②咨询本论文的其他作者或自己的导师等具有一定经验的专家。他们也许会有一些很好的建议。③浏览自己所引用的论文，看看是否有作者与你所开展的研究相似，可以考虑选择论文的第一或者通讯作者作为审稿人。在投稿阶段录入推荐人信息时，多需要提供其姓名、单位、邮箱及选择其作为审稿人的理由。除了提供推荐的审稿人，有个别期刊还要求提供需要回避的审稿人信息。

第3节　投稿后的工作

1. 投稿后，会发生什么

多数情况下，投稿后会出现以下三种情况：①"秒拒"；②格式审核不通过；③送外审。

（1）"秒拒"。

"秒拒"一般发生在投稿后的一到两天内（多数不超过一个星

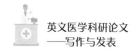

期）。投稿后，稿件会首先经过主编初审，如果他觉得该稿件与其期刊的收稿范围不一致或不属于其优先发表的范畴，则不考虑送外审而直接拒稿。下例就是我们既往投稿过程中遇到过的一个情形，如图7-2所示。

Subject: Beha____ ___ M__ine - Decision on Manuscript ID F __ 2020-0272

25-Sep-2020

Dear Dr I__ ba___:

I regret to inform you that I have now considered your paper submitted to B___ __ __ ___ ___cine but unfortunately have decided not to send it out for further review. We receive many more submissions to the journal than we are able to publish and thus the threshold for further evaluating manuscripts for possible publication is necessarily quite high. Unfortunately, your manuscript would likely be a low priority in terms of acceptance for publication because it is not within the scope of the journal and is not likely to be of interest to our readership who are largely behavioral medicine sleep providers and researchers. I would strongly urge you to consider the appropriateness of a journal and the topics of the articles published there before considering submitting your work elsewhere.

图7-2　"秒拒"邮件举例1

虽然不常见，但我们也遇到过如下被拒稿的情形：5月底投稿，之后未收到任何消息，直到9月初收到"被拒"邮件；且主编未将论文送外审，如图7-3所示。

Ref.: Ms. No. ___D-20-0P
Feasibility of s__p extensi__ __d its effe__ __io-me__ __ra__ter__ __tema__ __ and me__ __v__ of __ __ent__ __

Dear Dr. B___ ___,

Thank you for submitting your manuscript t___ ___ ___.

The Editorial Board has carefully considered the information presented in your work, but has decided not to send it out for peer review in its present format. You are however welcome to re-submit this manuscript as a Letter to the Editor. According to the Guide for Authors a Letter to the Editor may contain up to 300 words and five references.

The journal now receives many more papers than it can publish and many worthy articles have to be rejected. Therefore, we regret that we have to decline your current submission as it is.

图7-3　"被拒"邮件举例2

(2) 格式审核不通过。

某些期刊对所提交稿件的格式要求十分严格。有时候，稿件先要经过相关工作人员进行格式审查,然后再送给编辑审核。此时,作者需要针对该期刊要求修改的地方进行完善,然后再重新上传、提交稿件。如图 7-4 所示,我们既往的投稿过程中,遇到过稿件被返回进行微调。

05-Apr-2022

Dear Dr.

Your manuscript, 2-055 titled "Meas t p p es of t e S e 1 systematic review" has been temporarily unsubmitted as it needs minor formatting changes. These changes have been listed below.

Please make the necessary changes to your paper and then resubmit your manuscript by clicking 'Continue' (the original number assigned to your paper will then be retained). Please do not resubmit your amended paper as a new manuscript.

图7-4 稿件需要微调的邮件举例

(3) 送外审。

如果论文经过了编辑的初审,则会进入外审阶段。此阶段通常需要 2 个月左右,甚至更长。作者可登录投稿网站进行稿件状态查询。一般情况下,作者可以从投稿中心查阅到稿件目前所处状态。投稿完成后,稿件常见状态包括以下:①Submitted to journal:提示稿件已提交至期刊,等待被分配给相应的编辑。② Technical screening:期刊相关工作人员进行形式审查,确保该稿件符合期刊格式要求。如果不符合要求,则会被返回给作者,进行相应的修改。③With editor:提示稿件已送至编辑,编辑会审查该稿件内容是否符合期刊的范畴以及质量标准。如果符合,则送外审;若不符合,则拒稿。④Reviewer invited:提示编辑已经向审稿人发送审稿邀请,但是审稿人不一定接受邀请。⑤Under review:提示稿件处于外审阶段。⑥Required review completed:提示编辑已经收到各审稿人的意见,并对其进行汇总,送至主编做决定。⑦Decision in process:提示主编正在评估各审稿意见,并在做决定的过程中。⑧Revise or

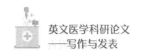
reject：修回或者拒稿。如果出现拒稿,多数情况下,也会向作者提供拒稿原因以及各审稿人给出的修改意见。对于修稿,后面将会详细介绍如何开展。

当然,不是每个期刊都会针对稿件设置这么多状态,而且其状态更新也可能没有那么及时。有时候,会遇到以下情况：投稿过了很久(例如,超过了该期刊一般的审稿周期),还未收到任何关于此稿件的消息。此时,可以登录作者中心,查阅稿件状态。如果处于"under review",那么还可以再等等,因为不是每个审稿人都会在规定的时间内完成审稿工作,毕竟审稿需要投入额外的时间去完成。如果处于"under review"之前的阶段(例如,"with editor"),那么,可以尝试给期刊发送邮件,询问一下稿件情况。有时候,也可能是作者中心稿件状态更新得不及时。

2. 如何给期刊发邮件,询问稿件状态

在给期刊发送邮件时,要注意邮件编写格式和内容。一般来说,邮件的主题需要包括稿号,还要体现出此封邮件的核心内容(例如,manuscript status inquiry)。如果从投稿平台的"作者中心(author center)"发送此邮件的话,邮件会自带稿号。以下是我们曾经给期刊办公室发送过的一封询问邮件以及期刊所给出的回复,如图 7 - 5 和图 7 - 6 所示。

Subject: Manuscript status inquiry

Dear Editorial staff,

Two weeks ago, we sent you an email to inquire about the status of our manuscript, which indicates "Required reviews completed". But, we did not get a response. Please excuse us for asking again whether you've reached a decision about our manuscript.

Thank you!

图 7 - 5　给期刊发邮件询问稿件状态

Thank you for your e-mail to the CIN editorial office. We apologize for the delay in the editorial review

process. Dr Nicoll was working off-site for an extended period of time. You should receive the results

of the review within the next 7 to 14 days.

If you have any questions, please e-mail.

图 7 - 6　期刊所给出的回复

第 4 节　稿件为何被拒

根据 *J Diabetes Complicat* 主编的反馈,其在做决定时,考虑的最主要因素是"该论文是否能够增加期刊对于读者的价值"。**首先**,创新性。许多研究重复既往已经开展过的研究,而未向读者展示新的内容。因此,作者在撰写论文之前,应该总结已知的并明确未知的。类似地,如果在新的人群中验证已经在其他人群中验证过的内容,其创新性也有限。**其次**,论文的主题(topic)、任务(mission)和研究结果所适用人群与目标期刊的一致性。例如,如果一个期刊是国际化期刊,而论文结果仅适用于某个国家,那么该论文就不适合投在此期刊中。当然,还要考虑论文对临床实践、未来研究及政策方面的影响。因此,主编会**优先考虑**以下论文:①可以保护及提高期刊的声誉;②内容具有创新性而不是简单的重复;③符合该期刊的任务、读者范围并能产生一定的影响(例如,临床实践、政策和科研)。论文能否得以接收,很大程度上与这些因素有关。知己知彼,方能百战不殆。了解背后的原因,有利于降低被拒稿的风险。

1. 论文被拒的常见原因有哪些

许多论文被拒的原因往往不止一个。多数国际期刊,尤其是领域内的顶级期刊,往往会收到许多高质量的稿件。但由于版面有限,该期刊只能接收属于其优先考虑范围的论文。例如,投稿于护理领域顶级期刊 *Int J Nurs Stud* 中的稿件,约 70% 会直接被主编拒稿。

(1) 未送外审直接被主编拒稿的原因。

1) 稿件不在期刊的刊发范围内。 明确稿件内容与期刊契合度的一种方法是浏览一下你的参考文献,看看所引用的论文是否发表在目标期刊或类似的期刊。如果没有,则很有可能表明你的稿件内容与期刊不一致。还有些期刊建议:可以在投稿前,先通过邮件联系主编,询问所投稿件是否适合该期刊。在询问时候,可以给主编发送论文的摘要,多数情况下主编会回复并给出自己的建议(可以投稿该刊或转投他刊)。这样的话,能够节省编辑和作者双方的时间。

2) 摘要和(或)贡献总结部分不具有说服力。 当编辑审稿时,首先看的就是摘要和(或)总结部分,如果无法很清晰地传达相关信息,吸引住编辑的眼球,则很有可能被拒稿。这一部分,要体现出本研究对于已有知识库的贡献,对未来研究、临床实践和政策等的启示。

3) 不能很清楚地阐明开展本研究的必要性。 这一点与论文的研究背景相关,也再次说明清晰的研究背景对于一篇论文的重要性。背景中,不仅要阐明已知的、未知的,更要体现本研究与既往研究的不同以及为什么这些不同很重要。*Int J Nurs Stud* 的主编提出,他在审稿时,十分注重研究的"创新性"和"贡献"。

4) 某国家的第一个研究。 多数期刊都是国际性期刊,其读者也来自全球各国。如果该研究唯一的新颖性是:它是某个国家的首个研究。那么,此稿件很可能被拒,因为它无法吸引来其他国家的读者。

5) 不容易被接收的文献类型: 概念分析(concept analysis)、integrative review、研究设计较弱的、pilot or feasibility study、量表研发相关论文。此类稿件很难发表在具有高影响力的期刊中。

(2) 审稿人拒稿的常见原因。

1) 语法存在大的问题。 有些作者提交的稿件在语法上存在很大的问题,而使得读者无法读懂作者想要表达的意思。因此,在投稿前,需要确保语法的准确性。

2) 论文撰写质量差。英文论文与中文论文的撰写在结构、风格、遣词上,均存在很大的差异。论文撰写质量可能决定论文的命运,因此,建议参考本书中前面介绍的要点,形成良好的书写习惯。

3) 研究汇报不完整。论文汇报不完整的话,审稿人就很难去判断研究的效度。对于有些编辑和审稿人,如果作者在稿件中遗漏了许多重要信息,则很有可能会直接拒稿,而不会要求作者再次澄清。这一点也再次说明按照汇报指南撰写论文的重要性。

4) 过度夸大结论。在撰写结论时,过度夸大研究的因果推断或影响力。常见的错误有:A 与 B 相关,但是给出的结论却是"A 影响 B";研究结果仅适用于某特定人群,但是给出的结论却延展到了所有人群。

2. 如何提高论文被接收的可能性

稿件提交后,主编是第一个对其做出评估的人,也许在几个小时后,他就决定拒稿或者将其分配给责任编辑;责任编辑再决定是否送外审。这一阶段其实非常重要,主编除了自己的全职工作,还要初审所有稿件,所以他们一般会根据自己的标准很快决定一篇稿件的去留。这些标准包括:该稿件是否能够达到责任编辑及审稿人的要求;该稿件潜在的影响力及被引的可能性(主编都希望发表会被别人引用的稿件)。根据 *J Adv Nurs* 主编的说法,他在审稿时,一般会参考以下标准:

(1) 稿件内容与期刊的一致度。投稿指南中,通常会明确该期刊的目的及范畴(aim and scope),可以看一下你的稿件内容是否与其相符合。此外,还可以大致浏览一下该期刊最近以及既往是否发表过类似主题的论文。这也是最重要的一点。如果契合度不高,建议不要投稿于该期刊。

（2）标题尽量简短，一般不超过 20 个单词。多数期刊都是国际性期刊，除非稿件内容是涉及全国范围的大型研究，否则尽量避免在标题中出现国家名称。避免在标题中使用 small, local, preliminary 等词。如果一个研究是严谨的，其大小并不是最重要的。当然，如果研究是一个 pilot or feasibility study，那么就需要在标题中体现出来，并按照相应的要求撰写该论文。

（3）**遵循格式要求及汇报指南**。不同类型的论文撰写时，需要遵循不同的汇报指南。常见的汇报指南有 PRISMA、CONSORT 等，论文的撰写需要符合该期刊所建议遵循的汇报指南。类似地，摘要格式也要按照投稿指南书写。如果摘要的格式都是错误的，那就说明作者没有仔细阅读投稿指南，很容易就被主编拒稿。

（4）**使用规范、正确的学术语言**。正确的语法是保证论文质量的基础，在撰写英文科研论文时，选择合适的词汇十分重要。例如，不可将具有因果推断含义的词汇与仅表示相关关系的词汇相混淆。前者常见的词汇包括 cause/induce/result in/lead to/contribute to，affect/influence/impact，modify，increase/elevate，decrease/reduce，improve；后者常见的词汇包括 associated with，related to，correlated with，linked to，predict，vary with，lower，higher。

第 5 节　稿件修回及接收

无论是写作新手还是有经验的学者，论文被拒都是不可避免的。面对被拒的论文，是直接投稿于新的期刊还是修改后再投，这是个值得思考的问题，尤其是对于缺乏投稿经验的新手而言。

针对以上问题，有两种情形，其处理方法也有所不同。第一种情形：稿件还未送外审，直接被拒。此时，作者可以根据新的目标期刊的投稿指南，对论文格式等进行修改。第二种情形：编辑或审稿人针对稿件提供了修改建议。此时,有些作者可能会直接忽略建议,将未经过修改的稿件投至新的期刊。但是,这种做法是十分不明智的:所投新期刊的审稿人可能与上一个拒稿期刊的审稿人是同一个(尤其是相关研究领域较小或较新时)。审稿是一个十分花费时间的事情,不考虑审稿人的建议,代表你十分不尊重他们的劳动成果。而且,新的审稿人可能提出与既往审稿人类似的建议。

拿到拒稿意见后,不要着急去修改。因为被拒稿后往往会出现沮丧、气愤等消极心理,影响对审稿意见的客观解读和判断。这时,不妨先把论文放几天甚至是更长时间,等到做好心理准备以后,再进行修改。在修改稿件时,并非一定要完全按照审稿人的意见和建议进行修改(有些可能并不合理)。但是,针对论文的条理性、准确性和格式等方面的建议,一般都需要进行修改。

1. 论文修回时的注意事项

有经验的作者会把编辑及审稿人的所有建议复制到一个 Word 文档中。每个问题单独列出,在进行回复时,从新的一段开始,并使用不同的字体将审稿人的问题及你的回复区分开来。**在对稿件进行修改时,切忌:**

(1) **针对审稿人提出的问题,未给出全面回答。**有时候,审稿人在提出的一个问题下面有几个小的分问题。此时,需要针对每个分问题逐条进行回复,而不是简单地概述。以下是我们既往投稿中遇到过的一种情况。虽然放在了一个问题下面,但是此审稿人其实是提出了两个问题/建议,如图 7 - 7 所示。针对此,我们给出了清晰、完整的回复,如图 7 - 8 所示。

(2) **针对审稿人提出的问题避而不谈。**有时候,作者没有读懂审稿人的建议;还有的时候,无法对审稿人提出的问题进行合理回复,有些作者就选择避而不答,这是在稿件修回过程中十分忌讳的一

Comment: It is not appropriate to group studies that measure food intake over a single meal with others that measured food intake over a day. In addition, the authors should not group studies that did not assess actual food intakes (such as those that used simulated tasks) with objective measures of food intake. These last studies could be used to support subjective assessments of appetite/hunger but not actual intakes.

图 7 - 7　审稿人的建议

Response: Thank you for your comments and suggestions. 1) We performed separate analyses for studies that measured energy intake over a single meal (n=3) and that measured energy intake over a day (n=8). 2) We excluded studies that did not use objective food intake from the meta-analysis and used them to support our findings on subjective hunger. After excluding these studies, subgroup analysis based on the type of intervention (PSR vs. TSD) was not applicable. Therefore, we deleted that part. We made corresponding changes in the results and discussion section as well as the figures. (p.8, p. 12, Fig. 3a and 3b, Table S2)

图 7 - 8　作者回复

种做法。因为，这会让审稿人觉得作者不尊重他。

（3）**过度不自信**。对于处于科研生涯初期的学者，在遇到审稿人提出的问题时，常会觉得不自信。最常见的一种表现是：在回复时候审稿人的问题时，喜欢使用"we are sorry . . ."。这种场合下，无须进行道歉，只要正面、客观地回答问题即可。

（4）**使用太多感谢**。表达对审稿人的感谢是应该的，但无须使用太多。有些作者喜欢在回复每个问题前，都给出"Thank you for your comments"，这个完全没有必要。

（5）**忽略重要细节**。每个期刊对于修改的要求不同，例如：有的要求使用"track change"来体现修改痕迹；有的要求在论文中对改动的地方使用不同的字体颜色或高亮来表示。多数情况下，都需要在回复中标注进行改动的页码（如示例 7 - 8 所示）。在修回过程中，要注意以上细节。

（6）**没有把握好修回的进度**。多数情况下，期刊会给作者 1～2

个月的时间,完成稿件的修回工作。根据论文是大修还是小修,每个人所需要的时间会有所不同。作者需要根据审稿人提出的问题,合理安排时间。有些作者有拖延症,习惯把工作拖到最后几天完成。但是,这会大大影响修回的质量。任何一个问题的回复,都需要时间和精力;尤其是一些基础论文,可能还需要补实验。如果没有安排好时间,就必须向编辑发邮件,要求其再宽限一些时间。当然,还有另一种常见的情形。有些作者喜欢很高效地把事情完成,可能不到一周(有时候甚至是 1~2 天)就完成了修回。如果是小修,这是很正常的。但是,如果是大修,则建议不要急于在短时间内就提交修回稿件。主要基于以下 3 点:①也许我们可以集中地回答完审稿人的问题,但是把修回的论文放几天之后,可能会有新的视角和想法,会提高修回的质量,修回的内容也需要反复的推敲和修改,这个过程是急不得的;②一般情况下,多需要把修回的论文和 response letter 发给其他作者(尤其是通讯作者)去阅读、进行完善,这也需要一段时间;③此外,欧美国家(许多期刊都是欧美国家承办)的工作风格/节奏比我们要慢很多,如果太快将稿件返修回去,有时候会让编辑觉得没有认真回答。

2. 如何针对审稿人的意见和建议给出合适的回复

对于大修的论文,面对审稿人的众多问题,可能会有很大的压力。此时,建议:①大致了解一下各审稿人的问题,然后根据自己的喜好有序回答。一部分作者习惯先回答简单的问题,把较难的问题放在最后。②在回答较难的问题时,最好计划逐步攻破(例如,每天回答两个)。这样,就不会显得困难太大而无法克服。③如果实在无法在规定的时间内完成修回,则需要在修回截止日期之前,提前向编辑发送邮件进行说明,要求其延长时间,多数情况下,这种请求都是被允许的。

此外,还需要注意,不是所有意见和建议都是合理且值得采纳的。如果你"不同意"某个建议,则可针对审稿人提出的问题,给出反驳(rebuttal)。在进行反驳时,一定不可找借口或狡辩,需要表示出对审稿人的尊重,并提出具体、客观、合理的原因(尽量有引文支持)。如图 7 - 9 所示,作者针对审稿人提出的问题进行了回复,同时针对今后可以开展的工作提出了建议。类似地,还有些情况,审稿人会要求你提供一些随访数据,但是本研究并未收集。此时,可以在 limitation 这一部分进行说明。通常情况下,审稿人都能够接受这样的回复,如图 7 - 10 所示。

Comment: In pregnancy, inflammation is thought to be involved in delivery timing. The authors do not discuss the salience of their investigation for birth timing or other adverse pregnancy outcomes (e.g., preeclampsia). Was this data collected?

Response: Yes. We collected this information. We agree that inflammation may be related to pregnancy outcomes, as supported by previous evidence. However, the main objective of this report was to investigate the associations between objective sleep and inflammation. Thus, we did not present data related to the outcomes. However, we added this information in the implication section. **(Page 14, 1ˢᵗ para)**

图 7 - 9   在"Implication"部分进行解释

Comments to the Author: Congratulations to the authors on such a splendid study. My only remark is that, *with such huge numbers, I would be interested in the outcome of PICC-RT patients vs. the no PICC-RT patients. If overall survival is impacted by the presence of PICC-RT, perhaps higher risk patients (identified by the risk factors described in this manuscript) should have this procedure denied.*

Response: We would like to thank the reviewer for this great suggestion. Unfortunately, in this retrospective study, we only extracted data related to the risk of PICC-RT. We did not have follow-up data, which has precluded us from conducting the survival analysis. In addition, examining the outcomes of PICC-RT seems like a different research question. However, we agree that comparing the outcomes (including survival data) of patients with PICC-RT and without PICC-RT is of great significance. We plan to pursue this line of investigation in future research. We also added this point in the implication section. **(Page 12-13)**

图 7 - 10   在"Limitation"部分进行说明

3. 论文修回时，如何撰写 Cover letter

多数情况下，在进行回复时，可以在 Response letter 的第一页，给出 Cover letter。Cover letter 里面需要包含论文标题、稿号等信息。图 7 - 11 是我们在撰写 Cover letter 时，常采用的格式：

Dear Prof. …,

Thank you very much for the review of our manuscript "*TITLE*" (*Manuscript ID...*). We greatly appreciate the constructive feedback from your reviewers and editorial staff. Your advice helped us improve this manuscript. Please forward our heartfelt thanks to these experts.

Based on your comments, we revised our manuscript and explain the revisions after each comment. All changes within the manuscript are highlighted in yellow.

We hope the changes are satisfactory. We look forward to hearing from you regarding our submission. We would be glad to respond to any further questions and comments that you may have.

Thank you!

Sincerely,

First or corresponding author

图 7 - 11　撰写 Cover letter 时常采用的格式

4. 论文接收后的工作

投稿过程中，最令人激动的时刻就是收到论文被接收的邮件。但是，论文被接收后，仍有重要的后续工作需要完成，例如：**校对稿件，签署版权转让书**。多数情况下，通讯作者会收到一封邮件，告知其如何完成稿件的校对和版权转让书的签署。在完成以上两项工作之前，论文不会被正式发表，也无法在数据库中检索到。值得注意的

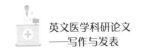

是,论文校对多数需要在 2～3 个工作日内完成,版权转让书也会要求尽快完成。因此,在收到论文被接收的邮件之后,要密切关注邮箱动态,以及时处理。

目前,多数期刊都会提供"OA"这一选项。OA 需要支付一定的费用,费用根据期刊不同而有所不同。OA 也有益处,例如:对于作者而言,其论文能更快、更全地被检索到(因为读者无须付费即可阅读到全文)。有些期刊需要通过个人或者单位付费后才能阅读并下载全文。通过 OA,可以提高论文的受众面。如果科研经费充足,又想要扩大论文的影响面,可以选择 OA。

第 **8** 章　论文发表涉及的伦理和学术规范

　　对于多数学者而言，发表论文的质量和数量是评价其学术成就的重要指标之一。发表论文对于个人的职业发展、申请基金、奖项及声誉都具有重要意义。与以上成果一并的便是责任，但是这一点却常常被忽略。为了避免学术不端，发表论文中常涉及的责任包括：保证所发表内容的准确性和可靠性、研究的开展遵循既定的伦理及指南、充分申报存在的利益冲突等。本章中，将通过回答以下问题，简要介绍论文发表过程中涉及的伦理和学术规范。

- 如何确定作者及作者顺序？
- 发表过程中有哪些常见的不端行为？
- 什么是利益冲突？

第1节　作者及作者顺序

　　一项研究或一篇论文多是团队合作的结果，往往会涉及多个贡献者（或作者）。就撰写论文而言，虽然默认为作者顺序代表其贡献度大小，但很多情况下，却很难界定，尤其是对于跨学科的大型研究。作者及作者顺序也是容易造成冲突的一个环节，因此，如何界定"作者"及确定作者顺序，均具有重要的现实意义。

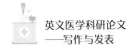
1. 什么是作者

ICMJE 对于"作者"的标准给出了明确规定。在同时满足以下 4 个条件的情况下，才能被列为作者出现在文中，否则，不能作为作者，仅可以被置于"致谢"部分。关于其具体说明，详见相关网站：

http://www. icmje. org/recommendations/browse/roles-and-responsibilities/defining-the-role-of-authors-and-contributors. html

• Substantial contributions to the conception or design of the work；or the acquisition，analysis，or interpretation of data for the work；AND【对论文的构思或设计做出实质性贡献；或对数据的获取、分析、解读做出实质性贡献】

• Drafting the work or revising it critically for important intellectual content；AND【起草论文或对论文的重要内容进行评判性修改】

• Final approval of the version to be published；AND【同意所发表的终版稿件】

• Agreement to be accountable for all aspects of the work in ensuring that questions related to the accuracy or integrity of any part of the work are appropriately investigated and resolved.【同意对论文各方面负责，以确保与各部分内容准确性和完整性有关的问题得到适当的调查和处理】

2. 几种常见的作者类型

在一篇论文中，目前关注较多的是**第一作者、通讯作者及 Senior author**。第一作者不言而喻，完成了本论文涉及的大部分工作，是该论文付出精力最多的人，是论文的主要撰写者。Corresponding author(通讯作者)通常是在所有作者同意的情况下,指定的一个作者。该作者负责论文投稿过程中及发表后与期刊联系等工作。一般情况下,项目负责人(即 PI)可以作为通讯作者。一篇论文可以没有 Senior author,但是必须要指定一个通讯作者。通讯作者可以是第一作者或者 Senior author,也可以是作者列表中的任意一名作者。Senior author 通常是最后一名作者,也许此作者在论文的撰写和研究开展过程中并未做太多工作,但他是该研究/论文的驱动力,起着统筹作用。此作者一般资历较深、获得了该项目的基金并指导其他作者工作。与欧美许多国家不同,我们目前的评价体系比较看重第一作者和通讯作者,而很少关注 Senior author。值得一提的是,基于目前的评价体系,不乏有人为了晋升而挂别人或者被挂为"共同第一"或"共同通讯"作者。有时候,甚至有多个"共同"。面对这样的窘境,个人、单位和国家需要共同努力。一方面,作者自身需要具有内在的约束力,遵循发表伦理。另一方面,单位和国家需要进一步优化现有的评价体系,为个人遵守发表伦理保驾护航。可喜的是,我国已经逐渐认识到了加强医学科研诚信建设、提高医学科研人员职业道德修养及预防科研不端行为的重要性。2021 年 2 月 19 日,国家卫生健康委、科技部、国家中医药管理局三部委结合相关法律法规修订了《医学科研诚信和相关行为规范》。该规范第 14 条要求,医学科研人员在发表论文或出版学术著作过程中,要遵守《发表学术论文"五不准"》和学术论文投稿、著作出版有关规定。论文、著作、专利等成果的署名应当按照对科研成果的贡献大小据实署名和排序,无实质学术贡献者不得"挂名"。

3. 常见问题

关于作者,现实中比较常见的问题包括"3G"作者:"Guest-author"、"Ghost-author"和"Gift-author"。这几种问题的出现受到个人、单位、地域和国家大环境的影响,会对科学界造成非常深远的不良后果。

Guest-author:指的是将比较有影响力的人(但是达不到作者的标准)加入文中,其目的是使得编辑、审稿人及读者更加偏向于相信此论文的质量。

Ghost-author:是指某人参与了论文的撰写,但是名字不在论文中。学生或处于职业生涯早期的科研人员可能会遇到此问题;常见的还有药物或器械公司人员,他们虽然对论文贡献很大,但是为了避免相关的利益冲突,而主动要求不将自己的名字放在论文中。

Gift-author:指的是将达不到作者标准的单位领导人(院长、系主任等)作为作者加入文中。

4. 一些建议

(1)尽早确定作者顺序:有学者建议所有作者应该在开始撰写论文之前,一起决定作者顺序,并根据实施过程中的实际情况进行调整。尽早地决定作者顺序,有利于避免冲突。在完成投稿后(尤其是稿件被接收后),尽量不要变更作者顺序。对于作者及作者顺序的任何变更都需要十分充分的理由,并获得所有作者的知情同意且签字。根据 COPE 指南,论文见刊后如果对作者进行更改,需要附有更正通知(correction 或 corrigendum)。严重的情况下,可能需要"撤回"此论文,这会严重影响该论文及其作者的信誉和可信度。既往文献也报道,在所有被撤回的论文中,有 6% 是由于"作者"相关问题引起的。当然,还有人在修回阶段添加新的作者。虽然作者可能给出了明确的原因,但是应该尽量避免此行为,因为这会让编辑及审稿人对于作者的可信度产生怀疑。从长远来看,可能会产生不良影响。

(2)明确作者贡献:目前,多数期刊要求在提交稿件时明确作者贡献。表 8-1 中,对 CRediT 中的"贡献者角色及其定义"进行了总

结。具体条目，可参考相关网站：https://www.elsevier.com/
authors/journal-authors/policies-and-ethics/credit-author-statement。

表 8 - 1　CRediT 中对于贡献者角色及其定义的介绍

贡献者角色	定　义
Conceptualization（构思）	Ideas; formulation or evolution of overarching research goals and aims
Methodology（方法学）	Development or design of methodology; creation of models
Software（软件）	Programming, software development; designing computer programs; implementation of the computer code and supporting algorithms; testing of existing code components
Validation（验证）	Verification, whether as a part of the activity or separate, of the overall replication/reproducibility of results/experiments and other research outputs
Formal analysis（数据分析）	Application of statistical, mathematical, computational, or other formal techniques to analyze or synthesize study data
Investigation（调查）	Conducting a research and investigation process, specifically performing the experiments, or data/evidence collection
Resources（资源）	Provision of study materials, reagents, materials, patients, laboratory samples, animals, instrumentation, computing resources, or other analysis tools

（续表）

贡献者角色	定　义
Data curation （获取数据）	Management activities to annotate （produce metadata）, scrub data and maintain research data （including software code, where it is necessary for interpreting the data itself） for initial use and later reuse
Writing-Original Draft （撰写初稿）	Preparation, creation and/or presentation of the published work, specifically writing the initial draft （including substantive translation）
Writing-Review & Editing （提供反馈）	Preparation, creation and/or presentation of the published work by those from the original research group, specifically critical review, commentary or revision – including pre-or post-publication stages
Visualization （可视化）	Preparation, creation and/or presentation of the published work, specifically visualization/ data presentation
Supervision （指导）	Oversight and leadership responsibility for the research activity planning and execution, including mentorship external to the core team
Project admini- stration （项目管理）	Management and coordination responsibility for the research activity planning and execution
Funding acquisition （获取基金）	Acquisition of the financial support for the project leading to this publication

第2节　常见学术不端行为

如同开展研究一样,论文发表过程中也涉及许多伦理问题。随着科学界对于学术诚信的要求越来越高以及检测学术不端行为的软件及网站的出现,越来越多的学术不端行为被曝光。在循证医学理念的指导下,临床决策(例如,制订诊疗方案及指南)多有赖于科学研究证据。在存在学术不端现象的情况下,作者可能会提供歪曲事实的数据或证据,进而误导同行科学家、卫生专业人员和决策者。此外,学术不端还会影响个人的声誉,有损作者所在单位甚至是国家在科学界的学术声誉和诚信度。因此,在实践过程中,每个人都应该严于律己,避免学术不端行为的发生。

1. 重复发表

根据 COPE (International Committee on Publication Ethics)的规定,重复发表被定义为"Major overlap/redundancy (i. e. based on same data with identical or very similar findings and/or evidence that authors have sought to hide redundancy, e. g. by changing title or author order or not citing previous papers)"。现实中,重复发表也并不少见。在发表论文前,首先要考虑的就是是否存在重复发表(duplication)。**根据既往发表的一篇论文,以下情况提示着可能存在重复发表**:①与既往论文中的研究假设相似;②研究的方法学基本一致;③研究结果基本一致;④几乎没有新的内容。当然,还有些时候,作者会对同一个研究进行二次分析(secondary analysis)。此时,需要在文中相应的地方,引用既往已经发表的论文;同时,在给编辑的 Cover letter 中,对此情况进行说明。下面以 *Nurs Res* 这一期刊

投稿指南中的相关内容进行解读。

(1)"论文的原创性"这一方面的要求。

● 所投稿件部分或全部内容未发表在其他地方(包括另一种语言):如果该稿件的摘要(abstract)已被发表或在某学术会议上进行了汇报,仍可考虑对其进行发表。

● 所投稿件不能已投稿于其他期刊。

● 每一篇论文都要对现有的文献/知识库做出独立贡献:所投稿件与既往论文存在重叠的话,需要说明该稿件有何新的贡献。多数期刊会使用"查重软件"对稿件进行查重。在某些情况下,可以允许基于同一研究项目进行"补充材料"或"二次分析"。此时,作者需要对编辑针对此情况进行说明,并向其提供既往论文的完整引文,以便其做出决定。如果在投稿阶段,未向编辑进行说明,则有可能直接被拒稿。

● 为了避免重复发表,还有学者建议:明确说明本论文与既往已发表论文相比较在研究问题上有何延伸;引用既往已发表的论文,并说明本论文是如何建立在既往论文基础上并充实相关研究结果的;明确说明本研究与既往已发表论文中重复的地方,例如研究方法。如图 8-1 所示,展示了我们在既往投稿中的一次类似经历。

This manuscript is a secondary analysis of data from a previously published study which was approved by the institutional review board of ??? The parent study examined the association between sleep and overall self-care, which answered a different research question (PMID: ???). We recently published a related paper (PMID: ???) that examined the relationship between fatigue, sleep disturbance, and eating style. In that paper, all the variables of interest were measured during the baseline interview and the instruments were different from the ones used in this paper. This paper adds to current literature by addressing the methodological limitations of the previous one. The manuscript described here has not been published previously and is not under consideration for publication elsewhere. All authors have approved the manuscript.

图 8-1　明确本论文和既往发表论文在研究问题上有何延伸

（2）香肠论文（salami publication）。

Salami publication 指的是不适当地将数据分割成最小的可发布单元（Salami publication refers to inappropriate fragmentation of data into the smallest publishable units）。根据近期发表的一项研究：常见的行为包括：①过度地将相互关联的个体暴露因素隔离开来进行验证；②研究问题密切相关，但却对不同的研究结果分别进行报道；③验后（post-hoc）亚组分析，例如：在同一队列中，对相同的暴露因素和结果根据亚组（subgroup）分别进行分析和报道。

目前，虽然学术界对于重复发表具有较一致的看法，但不同编辑对于香肠论文的界定尚未达成一致。为了避免作者发表香肠论文，有学者提出以下建议：①**督促作者**为了促进科学发展及临床实践而发表，对于同一研究收集到的不同数据，应力求提高发表论文的质量和全面性而减少发表论文数量。当确实需要发表多个论文时，也应尽量减少论文之间的重叠，并在 cover letter 中提及来自相同数据的已发表论文，同时说明本论文与既往论文有何区别。②**要求编辑**在投稿指南中，明确给出香肠论文的定义及检测此行为的方法，制定相关政策（例如，要求作者在投稿程中披露相关论文等），明确此行为的后果。③**提醒审稿人**在审稿过程中，需要注意是否存在香肠论文的迹象（例如，通过阅读研究方法可进行评估）。如果存在疑虑，应及时向编辑反馈。如果怀疑此行为，应及时进行汇报。④**完善学术奖励系统**：优化学术奖惩制度，强调论文质量而非数量；将其纳入学术评估系统中等。

2. 伪造数据、篡改数据、抄袭

（1）**伪造数据（data falsification）**：是指"编造数据并对其相关结果进行汇报"。常见的有：根本没有开展过相关研究，但却有研究结果；研究收集的样本量很小，但研究者在文中夸大样本量；将回顾性研究改成随机试验。现实中,很难识别这些问题。这些事件的调查非常具有挑战性,多需要举报人来揭穿。

(2) 篡改数据(data fabrication):是指"刻意操纵/篡改研究材料、设备或过程,更改或省略数据或结果,以至不能准确反映正确的研究记录"。此类问题很难确定,可以发生在不同层面,上至项目负责人,下至数据管理者。

(3) 抄袭(plagiarism):是指窃取别人的想法/文字/成果(复制、粘贴别人的论文)作为自己的,而未给予适当的引用。从期刊的角度出发,多数会使用查重软件,检验稿件是否存在抄袭(例如,iThenticate 或 CrossCheck)。如果检测出问题,轻则将稿件返回给作者修改重投;重则直接拒稿。从作者的角度出发,有不少人在撰写英文论文时,由于语言上存在障碍,选择复制前人的论文,尤其是研究背景和讨论部分。如果做得不合理,很容易造成抄袭。因此,在引用别人的论文时,应该避免大段地复制和粘贴既往文献,而是需要对其释义:使用自己的话对原文字进行转述,同时要引用该文献。此外,针对无法释义而必须使用作者原文的情况,应该使用双引号标注。

为了避免以上情况的发生,许多期刊目前都在投稿阶段要求作者提供 data availability 声明。同时要求研究的执行和汇报遵守特定的指南(例如,PRISMA、CONSORT 等)。对于系统文献综述和RCT,多数还要求:在项目开展前,对其进行**注册**。对于系统文献综述,可以在 PROSPERO 中对其进行注册(https://www.crd.york.ac.uk/PROSPERO/)。对于临床试验,可以在中国临床试验注册中心进行注册(http://www.chictr.org.cn/index.aspx)。

此外,还需注意所使用研究工具或者图片的版权。在研究开展前,就需要明确研究工具(问卷或量表)的版权并确定自己已获得使用该工具的许可。同时,在撰写论文时,要给出相应的引文。这样,在发表论文时,就不会涉及侵权。类似地,在撰写论文过程中,如果引用了既往已经发表的图片,需要获得版权所有者(出版机构)的许可。在使用某个研究工具之前,要确定该工具的版权(知识产权)所有者。如果该工具发表于某期刊或书籍中,则需要获得相应出版商的许可;如果该工具未发表于期刊论文或书籍,则可考虑与作者联系并获得许可。如果作者更改了联系方式,可搜索其最近发表的论文进而获取其新的联系方式。有些作者会将其研究工具发表在其教师网页或专业网站上,以获得广泛的使用许可。还有些作者可能会对研究工具的使用进行一些限制,例如不能更改条目的格式或措辞。如果研究人员已竭尽全力,但仍无法与版权所有者取得联系,则可考虑合理使用此工具。理想情况下,应与权威的版权来源(例如:图书馆馆员)共同做出决定。无论是何种情况,应对自己在寻求许可过程中所做出的努力和决策过程进行记录,以备将来出现问题时使用。

3. 学术不端的后果

以上学术不端行为会在多个层面上造成不良影响。**首先**,对于作者个人而言,如果被查出存在以上行为,可能会受到不同程度的处分,包括:收到期刊编辑或单位的警告、撤稿、撤回资助基金,作者或其所在单位被相关期刊或者出版社列入黑名单,无法申请基金课题,被吊销奖项,被解雇,受到法律制裁等。**其次**,如果以上不端行为未被发现,错误的数据及研究发现可能会将研究领域推向错误的方向,并浪费科研工作者的时间、精力和资金。类似地,错误的数据还可能为临床实践或者医学指南提供错误证据,进而可能对患者造成伤害。**再者**,由于科研基金和论文版面有限,认真做研究的学者可能在不同程度上被学术不规范者"击败",导致资源没有得到合理使用或者浪费大量的资源。

虽然每位学者都应该遵守学术规范,但是每天被撤回的论文仍

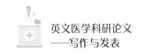

层出不穷。Retraction Watch(https://retractionwatch.com/)上,对被撤回的论文进行着实时更新。2018 年的一篇报道,对被撤稿的论文进行了分析,发现造成撤稿的主要原因有:学术不端(占 51%)、错误(占 14%)及重复发表(占 13%)。此外,针对撤稿要求提出方的多选调查结果为:期刊主编(占 59%)、作者(占 28%)、出版社(占 16%)、单位(占 6%)。

预防学术不端,需要国家、单位及科研人员(包括学生)的共同努力。虽然个人应严格遵守学术规范,但是单位也起着至关重要的作用。为了帮助个人预防以上不良学术行为的发生,单位可以与科研人员及学生分享最新的学术不端案例,设置相应的课程或作业,进而加强个人对于学术规范的认识。单位还应鼓励科研人员针对学术规范或者不端行为存在的疑问进行开诚布公的沟通和交流。在国家层面,出台强有力的政策也是预防学术不端的重要保障。例如,《关于进一步加强科研诚信建设的若干意见》《学位论文作假行为处理办法》《高等学校预防与处理学术不端行为办法》《医学科研诚信和相关行为规范》等一系列政策的制定与修订,为抵制学术不端行为、维护良好的学术生态环境提供了政策保障。

第 3 节　利益冲突

道德诚信是维护健康和纯洁学术环境的重要基础。提高论文发表透明度有利于研究者们更有效地分享研究资讯、加深对研究本身和学术知识的理解。为提高发表透明度,研究者有义务披露与研究相关的所有利益冲突并避免潜在问题。利益冲突披露(disclosure)是学术伦理的一种常见要求,也是科研人员对自身行为规范的良心约束。然而,不同期刊对利益冲突的管理政策要求不一,很多研究者对利益冲突的陈述也千差万别。因此,有必要深入了解利益冲突,进而为读者提供透明度更高的论文。

1. 利益冲突

"利益冲突"一词由来已久,从字面意义上判断,它是指不同利益主体之间的争夺和竞争。本文主要关注期刊论文发表过程中的利益冲突。依据 ICMJE 的定义,利益冲突是指作者、审稿人或期刊主编允许自我相关利益影响决策的情况(A conflict of interest occurs when an author, reviewer, or editor allows a self-interest to influence judgment)。利益冲突中牵涉到的利益可能是经济的、专业的、学术的、伦理的、政治的或个人的。从出版伦理委员会(COPE)官方网站展示的案例可以看出,实际或潜在影响论文学术观点及发表的利益冲突不但包括作者本人的利益冲突,还包括其他相关人员或相关方的利益冲突,如审稿人、编委会成员、期刊、研究机构、资助方,甚至是读者本人。一般来说,在所有这些利益冲突中,论文作者的利益冲突最为突出和受到关注。

需要强调的是,利益冲突可能是潜在的,也可能是实际发生的。利益冲突并非必然造成或引发严重的不良后果。研究者有必要在论文发表的过程中披露科研活动中可能的相关利益冲突,提高论文透明度,便于读者知晓全貌和做出判断。

2. 期刊论文发表常见的利益冲突类型

利益冲突的类型因划分标准不同而有差异:按利益冲突涉及的对象可以分为涉及作者的利益冲突、涉及审稿人的利益冲突、涉及编辑团队的利益冲突、涉及期刊的利益冲突、涉及资助方的利益冲突;按照利益冲突的内容,可以将期刊论文发表过程中的利益冲突分为经济利益冲突、关系利益冲突、竞争利益冲突、私隙利益冲突、良心利

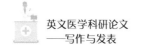
益冲突。本文主要介绍后者。

（1）**经济利益冲突**：在科研计划、研究实施、论文撰写、同行评议、论文发表的全过程中存在的经济利益上的冲突。科研过程中牵涉到的经济利益有多种形式，如企业资助的经费、企业顾问、股权所有权、雇佣合同、各种形式的津贴、咨询费、投资、储蓄、非货币形式的有价物品（馈赠或礼品）等。

（2）**关系利益冲突**：科研论文发表过程中，研究团队成员与审稿人或期刊编委会成员存在特殊的人际关系，如亲戚、同事、上下级、朋友等。更广义的关系甚至可以是非私人的关系，如审稿人或编委会成员与其曾任职机构之间的关系、学术合作关系等。

（3）**竞争利益冲突**：在科研活动中，研究团队与审稿人存在竞争关系，如申请同一个领域内的经费、同一研究领域内相近的课题研究或同一工作单位晋升或待遇等方面的竞争等。

（4）**私隙利益冲突**：科研论文发表过程中，研究团队成员与审稿人或期刊编委会成员存在个人恩怨、学术观点迥异或有其他私人感情问题等。

（5）**良心利益冲突**：由于受到政治、伦理、宗教等因素的影响，审稿人或期刊编委会成员对研究团队成员或研究课题本身存在偏见，从而影响到对研究或论文的科学公正判断，这些冲突统称为良心利益冲突。如某个审稿人可能对本身有争议的话题有自己的判断和情感，这些判断和情感会使他对相关话题的稿件持有偏见或偏袒，而不是依据论文的学术价值给出公正判断。

在以上 5 种利益冲突中，经济利益冲突最易确认和判断，其他内容的利益冲突需要论文作者或相关利益方主动揭露，呈现科研活动全貌，提升研究的透明度。

3. 期刊利益冲突的披露规范

近些年来,为提高论文发表的透明度,论文发表过程中的利益冲突问题受到了越来越多期刊的重视,绝大多数期刊均有明确的利益冲突披露的规范和要求。一项对护理类国际期刊利益冲突相关披露规范和管理的研究显示,在被调查的 116 种护理类国际期刊中,97.4%的护理期刊对论文作者有明确的利益冲突披露要求和原则,然而仅有 36.2%的期刊对审稿人有利益冲突披露要求,31.9%的期刊对其主编或编委会成员有利益冲突披露要求,这也说明论文作者的利益冲突最为突出和受人关注。

投稿过程中,论文作者应仔细研读期刊对于利益冲突披露的要求和规范,主动披露科研过程和论文投稿过程中可能存在的利益冲突。本文以 ICMJE 的披露表格(ICMJE Disclosure Form)为例,呈现论文发表过程中利益冲突的披露规范。

ICMJE 的披露表格中,论文作者应在表格中填写日期、作者姓名、论文题目以及论文编号(如果有)。表格列出需要披露的 13 种情况,除了第一种情况没有时间限制外,其余的利益冲突披露的时间界定均为过去的 36 个月内。这 13 种情况包括:①论文研究收到的所有资助(如资金、实验材料、医学写作、文章发表费用等),此条没有时间限制;②从任何一个实体获得的基金或合同;③版税或执照;④咨询费;⑤因演讲、报告、文章撰写或其他教育活动而获得的收入或酬金;⑥专家咨询费;⑦参会或差旅资助;⑧计划中、申请中或已经批准的专利;⑨参与了某个数据安全监管委员会或咨询会;⑩在其他委员会、社会组织、咨询委员会等有领导职务或受人委托(无论有偿或无偿);⑪股票或股票期权;⑫仪器、材料、药物、论文写作、礼物或其他服务的接收方;⑬其他经济或非经济的利益。

论文作者要对每个情况进行回答,列出所有相关的可能影响论文内容的利益方和非利益方,供其他读者了解和判断。ICMJE 也指出,利益冲突披露代表着提升发表的透明度而非引入偏见。ICMJE 表格填写完成后,可以在各个期刊的投稿系统内上传至期刊,作为利益冲突声明。然而,并非所有期刊均要求提供 ICMJE 披露表格,论文作者在投稿时,需阅读期刊对于利益冲突披露的要求和规范,并按照要求对论文可能牵涉的利益冲突进行陈述。

参考文献

[1] ZWAKENBERG SR, DE JONG PA, BARTSTRA JW, et al. The effect of menaquinone-7 supplementation on vascular calcification in patients with diabetes: A randomized, double-blind, placebo-controlled trial [J]. Am J Clin Nutr. 2019;110(4): 883 - 890.

[2] ZITSER J, ANATÜRK M, ZSOLDOS E, et al. Sleep duration over 28 years, cognition, gray matter volume, and white matter microstructure: A prospective cohort study [J]. Sleep. 2020;43(5).

[3] KIM EK, KWAK SH, JUNG HS, et al. The effect of a smartphone-based, patient-centered diabetes care system in patients with type 2 diabetes: A randomized, controlled trial for 24 weeks [J]. Diabetes Care. 2019;42(1): 3 - 9.

[4] IOVINO P, DE MARIA M, MATARESE M, et al. Depression and self-care in older adults with multiple chronic conditions: A multivariate analysis [J]. J Adv Nurs. 2020;76(7): 1668 - 1678.

[5] CHEN ZZ, LIU J, MORNINGSTAR J, et al. Metabolite profiles of incident diabetes and heterogeneity of treatment effect in the Diabetes Prevention Program [J]. Diabetes. 2019;68(12): 2337 - 2349.

[6] CHANG CF, YEH MK, CHIEN WC, et al. Interactions between psychiatric and physical disorders and their effects on the risks of suicide: A nested case-control study [J]. Ann N Y Acad Sci. 2020;1462(1): 79 - 91.

[7] BLANKEN TF, BORSBOOM D, PENNINX BW, et al. Network outcome analysis identifies difficulty initiating sleep as a primary target for prevention of depression: A 6-year prospective study [J]. Sleep. 2020;43(5).

[8] KLOOS N, DROSSAERT CHC, BOHLMEIJER ET, et al. Online positive psychology intervention for nursing home staff: A cluster-

randomized controlled feasibility trial of effectiveness and acceptability [J]. Int J Nurs Stud. 2019;98: 48 – 56.

[9] QI J, XU J, LI BZ, et al. The evaluation of sleep disturbances for Chinese frontline medical workers under the outbreak of COVID – 19 [J]. Sleep Med. 2020;72: 1 – 4.

[10] BAGNASCO A, DASSO N, ROSSI S, et al. A cross-sectional multisite exploration of Italian paediatric nurses' reported burnout and its relationship to perceptions of clinical safety and adverse events using the RN4CAST@IT-Ped [J]. J Adv Nurs. 2020.

[11] DE LIMA LOPES J, NEGRÃO BAPTISTA RC, TAKAO LOPES C, et al. Efficacy of a video during bed bath simulation on improving the performance of psychomotor skills of nursing undergraduates: A randomized clinical trial [J]. Int J Nurs Stud. 2019;99: 103333.

[12] IOVINO P, LYONS KS, DE MARIA M, et al. Patient and caregiver contributions to self-care in multiple chronic conditions: A multilevel modelling analysis [J]. Int J Nurs Stud. 2021;116: 103574.

[13] ORGAMBÍDEZ A, ALMEIDA H. Exploring the link between structural empowerment and job satisfaction through the mediating effect of role stress: A cross-sectional questionnaire study [J]. Int J Nurs Stud. 2020; 109: 103672.

[14] SHIMOURA K, IIJIMA H, SUZUKI Y, et al. Immediate effects of transcutaneous electrical nerve stimulation on pain and physical performance in individuals with preradiographic knee osteoarthritis: A randomized controlled trial [J]. Arch Phys Med Rehabil. 2019;100(2): 300 – 306. e301.

[15] SCHMIDT JJ, LUECK C, ZIESING S, et al. Clinical course, treatment and outcome of Pneumocystis pneumonia in immunocompromised adults: A retrospective analysis over 17 years [J]. Critical care (London, England). 2018;22(1): 307.

[16] KIRYU S, YASAKA K, AKAI H, et al. Deep learning to differentiate parkinsonian disorders separately using single midsagittal MR imaging: A proof of concept study [J]. Eur Radiol. 2019;29(12): 6891 – 6899.

[17] KYLE SD, HURRY MED, EMSLEY R, et al. The effects of digital cognitive behavioral therapy for insomnia on cognitive function: A randomized controlled trial [J]. Sleep. 2020;43(9).

[18] ZHU B, QUINN L, KAPELLA MC, et al. Relationship between sleep disturbance and self-care in adults with type 2 diabetes [J]. Acta Diabetol. 2018;55(9): 963 – 970.

[19] PYATAK EA, CARANDANG K, VIGEN CLP, et al. Occupational therapy intervention improves glycemic control and quality of life among young adults with diabetes: The Resilient, Empowered, Active Living with Diabetes (REAL Diabetes) randomized controlled trial [J]. Diabetes Care. 2018;41(4): 696 – 704.

[20] MAGNUSON A, LEI L, GILMORE N, et al. Longitudinal relationship between frailty and cognition in patients 50 years and older with breast cancer [J]. J Am Geriatr Soc. 2019;67(5): 928 – 936.

[21] SÁNCHEZ-DE-LA-TORRE M, SÁNCHEZ-DE-LA-TORRE A, BERTRAN S, et al. Effect of obstructive sleep apnoea and its treatment with continuous positive airway pressure on the prevalence of cardiovascular events in patients with acute coronary syndrome (ISAACC study): A randomised controlled trial [J]. Lancet Respir Med. 2020;8(4): 359 – 367.

[22] HIGGINS JPT, SAVOVIC J, PAGE MJ, et al. Assessing risk of bias in a randomized trial [M]//HIGGINS J P T, THOMAS J, CHANDLER J, et al. Cochrane Handbook for Systematic Reviews of Interventions version 6. 3 (updated February 2022). Cochrane; 2022.

[23] BROWN J, CRAWFORD TJ, DATTA S, et al. Oral contraceptives for pain associated with endometriosis [J]. Cochrane Database Syst Rev. 2018;5(5): Cd001019.

[24] SHEN W, GUAN YY, WU RM, et al. Protective effects of Wang-Bi tablet on bone destruction in collagen-induced arthritis by regulating osteoclast-osteoblast functions [J]. J Ethnopharmacol. 2019; 238: 111861.

[25] LI D, LIU J, GUO B, et al. Osteoclast-derived exosomal miR – 214 – 3p inhibits osteoblastic bone formation [J]. Nat Commun. 2016;7: 10872.

[26] ZIEGLER CGK, ALLON SJ, NYQUIST SK, et al. SARS-CoV-2 Receptor ACE2 is an interferon-stimulated gene in human airway epithelial cells and is detected in specific cell subsets across Tissues [J]. Cell. 2020; 181(5): 1016 – 1035. e19.

[27] BENTHEM SD, SKELIN I, MOSELEY SC, et al. Impaired hippocampal-cortical interactions during sleep in a mouse model of

Alzheimer's disease [J]. Curr Biol, 2020;30(13): 2588 – 2601. e5.

[28] MENG F, LI Z, ZHANG Z, et al. MicroRNA – 193b – 3p regulates chondrogenesis and chondrocyte metabolism by targeting HDAC3 [J]. Theranostics. 2018;8(10): 2862 – 2883.

[29] GREENBLATT HM, ROZENBERG H, DAITCHMAN D, et al. Does PCNA diffusion on DNA follow a rotation-coupled translation mechanism [J]? Nat Commun. 2020;11(1): 5000.

[30] OH J, MATKOVICH SJ, RIEK AE, et al. Macrophage secretion of miR – 106b – 5p causes renin-dependent hypertension [J]. Nat Commun. 2020;11(1): 4798.

[31] SU W, LIU G, LIU X, et al. Angiogenesis stimulated by elevated PDGF – BB in subchondral bone contributes to osteoarthritis development [J]. JCI Insight. 2020;5(8).

[32] LI M, FU X, GAO H, et al. Regulation of an osteon-like concentric microgrooved surface on osteogenesis and osteoclastogenesis [J]. Biomaterials. 2019;216: 119269.

[33] FLORENCIO-SILVA R, SASSO GRS, SASSO-CERRI E, et al. Effects of estrogen status in osteocyte autophagy and its relation to osteocyte viability in alveolar process of ovariectomized rats [J]. Biomed Pharmacother, 2018;98: 406 – 415.

[34] DAY RE, SAHOTA P, CHRISTIAN MS. Effective implementation of primary school-based healthy lifestyle programmes: A qualitative study of views of school staff [J]. BMC Public Health. 2019;19(1): 1239.

[35] GUNAWAN J, AUNGSUROCH Y, MARZILLI C, et al. A phenomenological study of the lived experience of nurses in the battle of COVID – 19 [J]. Nurs Outlook. 2021;69(4): 652 – 659.

[36] LIVINGSTON LA, SHAH P, HAPPÉ F. Compensatory strategies below the behavioural surface in autism: A qualitative study [J]. Lancet Psychiatry. 2019;6(9): 766 – 777.

[37] MANTOVAN F, MUZZANA C, SCHUBERT M, et al. "It's about how we do it, not if we do it". Nurses' experiences with implicit rationing of nursing care in acute care hospitals: A descriptive qualitative study [J]. Int J Nurs Stud. 2020;109: 103688.

[38] TKATCH R, MUSICH S, MACLEOD S, et al. A qualitative study to examine older adults' perceptions of health: Keys to aging successfully

[J]. Geriatr Nurs. 2017;38(6): 485 - 490.

[39] LU Q, MÅRTENSSON J, ZHAO Y, et al. Living on the edge: Family caregivers' experiences of caring for post-stroke family members in China: A qualitative study [J]. Int J Nurs Stud. 2019;94: 1 - 8.

[40] MARGARITI C, GANNON KN, WALSH JJ, et al. GP experience and understandings of providing follow-up care in prostate cancer survivors in England [J]. Health Soc Care Community. 2020;28(5): 1468 - 1478.

[41] NTOIMO LFC, OKONOFUA FE, IGBOIN B, et al. Why rural women do not use primary health centres for pregnancy care: Evidence from a qualitative study in Nigeria [J]. BMC Pregnancy Childbirth. 2019;19(1): 277.

[42] VAN CORVEN CTM, BIELDERMAN A, WIJNEN M, et al. Defining empowerment for older people living with dementia from multiple perspectives: A qualitative study [J]. Int J Nurs Stud. 2021; 114: 103823.

[43] SUTER J, KOWALSKI T, ANAYA-MONTES M, et al. The impact of moving to a 12 h shift pattern on employee wellbeing: A qualitative study in an acute mental health setting [J]. Int J Nurs Stud. 2020;112: 103699.

[44] HANNA A, YAEL EM, HADASSA L, et al. "It's up to me with a little support"-Adherence after myocardial infarction: A qualitative study [J]. Int J Nurs Stud. 2020;101: 103416.

[45] PALESE A, GNECH D, PITTINO D, et al. Non-nursing tasks as experienced by nursing students: Findings from a phenomenological interpretative study [J]. Nurse Educ Today. 2019;76: 234 - 241.

[46] ZHANG J, LEE DTF. Meaning in stroke family caregiving in China: A phenomenological study [J]. J Fam Nurs. 2019;25(2): 260 - 286.

[47] ROBERTSEN IL, SKÄR L. Oncology nurses' experiences of meeting with men with cancer-related fatigue: A qualitative study [J]. Scand J Caring Sci. 2021;35(1): 252 - 259.

[48] FINDLEY A, SMITH DM, HESKETH K, et al. Exploring womens' experiences and decision making about physical activity during pregnancy and following birth: A qualitative study [J]. BMC Pregnancy Childbirth. 2020;20(1): 54.

[49] ANDREWS H, TIERNEY S, SEERS K. Needing permission: The experience of self-care and self-compassion in nursing: A constructivist

grounded theory study [J]. Int J Nurs Stud. 2020;101: 103436.

[50] BELOGIANNI K, BALDWIN C. Types of interventions targeting dietary, physical activity, and weight-related outcomes among university students: A systematic review of systematic reviews [J]. Adv Nutr. 2019;10(5): 848 - 863.

[51] SCOTT H, LACK L, LOVATO N. A systematic review of the accuracy of sleep wearable devices for estimating sleep onset [J]. Sleep Med Rev. 2020;49: 101227.

[52] ALIMORADI Z, LIN CY, BROSTRÖM A, et al. Internet addiction and sleep problems: A systematic review and meta-analysis [J]. Sleep Med Rev. 2019;47: 51 - 61.

[53] ALDRIDGE RW, NELLUMS LB, BARTLETT S, et al. Global patterns of mortality in international migrants: A systematic review and meta-analysis [J]. Lancet. 2018;392(10164): 2553 - 2566.

[54] MOOSAVIAN SP, ARAB A, PAKNAHAD Z. The effect of a Mediterranean diet on metabolic parameters in patients with non-alcoholic fatty liver disease: A systematic review of randomized controlled trials [J]. Clin Nutr ESPEN. 2020;35: 40 - 46.

[55] ZHU B, SHI C, PARK CG, et al. Effects of sleep restriction on metabolism-related parameters in healthy adults: A comprehensive review and meta-analysis of randomized controlled trials [J]. Sleep Med Rev. 2019;45: 18 - 30.

[56] JONES RN, CIZGINER S, PAVLECH L, et al. Assessment of instruments for measurement of delirium severity: A systematic review [J]. JAMA Intern Med. 2019;179(2): 231 - 239.

[57] MUÑOZ BALBONTÍN Y, STEWART D, SHETTY A, et al. Herbal medicinal product use during pregnancy and the postnatal period: A systematic review [J]. Obstet Gynecol. 2019;133(5): 920 - 932.

[58] HUNTER H, LOVEGROVE C, HAAS B, et al. Experiences of people with Parkinson's disease and their views on physical activity interventions: A qualitative systematic review [J]. JBI Database Syst Rev Implement Rep. 2019;17(4): 548 - 613.

[59] KANESARAJAH J, WALLER M, WHITTY JA, et al. Multimorbidity and quality of life at mid-life: A systematic review of general population studies [J]. Maturitas. 2018;109: 53 - 62.

［60］ KARKOU V，AITHAL S，ZUBALA A，et al. Effectiveness of dance movement therapy in the treatment of adults with depression：A systematic review with meta-analyses ［J］. Front Psychol. 2019;10：936.

［61］ HARRIS JD，QUATMAN CE，MANRING MM，et al. How to write a systematic review ［J］. Am J Sports Med. 2014;42(11)：2761 - 2768.

［62］ AMERICAN PSYCHOLOGICAL ASSOCIATION. Publication Manual of the American Psychological Association ［M］. 7th ed. ，American Psychological Association. 2020.

［63］ ZHU B，BRONAS UG，CARLEY DW，et al. Relationships between objective sleep parameters and inflammatory biomarkers in pregnancy ［J］. Ann N Y Acad Sci. 2020;1473(1)：62 - 73.

［64］ ZHU B，YIN Y，SHI C，et al. Feasibility of sleep extension and its effect on cardiometabolic parameters in free-living settings：A systematic review and meta-analysis of experimental studies ［J］. Eur J Cardiovasc Nurs. 2022;21(1)：9 - 25.

［65］ SPURLOCK JR. D. Using existing research instruments：Copyright，permission，and fair use ［J］. Nurse Author Ed. 2019;29(1)：1 - 6.

［66］ DING D，NGUYEN B，GEBEL K，et al. Duplicate and salami publication：A prevalence study of journal policies ［J］. Int J Epidemiol. 2020;49(1)： 281 - 288.

［67］ MISRA DP，RAVINDRAN V，AGARWAL V. Integrity of authorship and peer review practices：Challenges and opportunities for improvement ［J］. J Korean Med Sci. 2018;33(46)：e287.

［68］ ZIETMAN AL. Falsification，fabrication，and plagiarism：The unholy trinity of scientific writing ［J］. Int J Radiat Oncol Biol Phys. 2013;87(2)： 225 - 227.

［69］ WANG B，LAI J，YAN X，et al. Exploring the characteristics，global distribution and reasons for retraction of published articles involving human research participants：A literature survey ［J］. Eur J Intern Med. 2020;78： 145 - 146.

［70］ ANNANE D，LEROLLE N，MEURIS S，et al. Academic conflict of interest ［J］. Intensive Care Med. 2019;45(1)：13 - 20.

［71］ BARNSTEINER J，SHAWN KENNEDY M，FLANAGIN A，et al. Nursing journal policies on disclosure and management of conflicts of interest ［J］. J Nurs Scholarsh. 2020;52(6)：680 - 687.

[72] GRUNDY Q, DUNN AG, BERO L. Improving researchers' conflict of interest declarations [J]. BMJ. 2020;368: m422.

[73] 黄小茹. 学术期刊论文发表过程中的利益冲突及其处理[J]. 编辑学报. 2013;2: 161 - 164.

[74] THAPA DK, VISENTIN DC, HUNT GE, et al. Being honest with causal language in writing for publication [J]. J Adv Nurs. 2020;76(6): 1285 - 1288.

[75] KAREN HOLLAND, ROGER WATSON. Writing for Publication in Nursing and Healthcare: Getting it Right [M]. 2nd ed. USA: John Wiley & Sons Ltd, 2021.

[76] CARTER-TEMPLETON H. Writing productivity strategies [J]. Nurse Author Ed. 2021;31(2): 33 - 35.

[77] BAVDEKAR SB, TULLU MS. Research publications for academic career advancement: An idea whose time has come. But is this the right way [J]. J Postgrad Med. 2016;62(1): 1 - 3.

[78] MABVUURE NT. Twelve tips for introducing students to research and publishing: A medical student's perspective [J]. Med Teach. 2012; 34 (9): 705 - 709.

[79] MUNN Z, PETERS MDJ, STERN C, et al. Systematic review or scoping review? Guidance for authors when choosing between a systematic or scoping review approach [J]. BMC Med Res Methodol. 2018;18(1): 143.

[80] BHARGAVA P, AGRAWAL G. From the editor's desk: A systematic guide to revising a manuscript [J]. Radiol Case Rep. 2013;8(1): 824.

[81] GROSS C. Scientific Misconduct [J]. Annu Rev Psychol. 2016;67: 693 - 711.

[82] GREY A, BOLLAND MJ, AVENELL A, et al. Check for publication integrity before misconduct [J]. Nature. 2020;577(7789): 167 - 169.

[83] GRANT MJ, BOOTH A. A typology of reviews: An analysis of 14 review types and associated methodologies [J]. Health Info Libr J. 2009; 26(2): 91 - 108.

[84] KOTTNER J, NORMAN I. How to peer review and revise manuscripts submitted for publication in academic nursing journals [J]. Int J Nurs Stud. 2016;64: A1 - A3.

[85] CONN VS. Should authors revise a rejected manuscript prior to submitting to a new journal [J]. West J Nurs Res. 2014; 36 (8):

955 - 956.

[86] PHILLIPPI JC, LIKIS FE, TILDEN EL. Authorship grids: Practical tools to facilitate collaboration and ethical publication [J]. Res Nurs Health. 2018;41(2): 195 - 208.

[87] MASTEN Y, ASHCRAFT A. Due diligence in the open-access explosion era: Choosing a reputable journal for publication [J]. FEMS Microbiol Lett. 2017;364(21).

[88] WATSON R. Which articles get published and why [J]? J Adv Nurs. 2019;75(6): 1149 - 1150.

[89] WALLACE MB, BOWMAN D, HAMILTON-GIBBS H, et al. Ethics in publication, part 2: Duplicate publishing, salami slicing, and large retrospective multicenter case series [J]. Gastrointest Endosc. 2018; 87 (5): 1335 - 1337.

[90] STOCKS A, SIMCOE D, TOROSER D, et al. Substantial contribution and accountability: Best authorship practices for medical writers in biomedical publications [J]. Curr Med Res Opin. 2018; 34 (6): 1163 - 1168.

[91] AROMATARIS E, FERNANDEZ R, GODFREY CM, et al. Summarizing systematic reviews: Methodological development, conduct and reporting of an umbrella review approach [J]. Int J Evid Based Healthc. 2015;13(3): 132 - 140.

[92] SMITH E, WILLIAMS-JONES B. Authorship and responsibility in health sciences research: A review of procedures for fairly allocating authorship in multi-author studies [J]. Sci Eng Ethic. 2012;18(2): 199 - 212.

[93] GRIFFITHS P, NORMAN I. Why was my paper rejected? Editors' reflections on common issues which influence decisions to reject papers submitted for publication in academic nursing journals [J]. Int J Nurs Stud. 2016;57: A1 - A4.

[94] MCCANN TV, POLACSEK M. Addressing the vexed issue of authorship and author order: A discussion paper [J]. J Adv Nurs. 2018,74(9): 2064 - 2074.

[95] SHAMSEER L, DAVID MOHER. Planning a systematic review? Think protocols [EB/OL]. (2015 - 01 - 05)[2021 - 11 - 01]. https://blogs.biomedcentral.com/bmcblog/2015/01/05/planning-a-systematic-review-think-protocols/

网络资源

1. 不同类型论文汇报指南汇总：https://www.equator-network.org/
2. CONSORT 汇报指南：https://www.equator-network.org/reporting-guidelines/consort/
3. STROBE 汇报指南：https://www.equator-network.org/reporting-guidelines/strobe/
4. CONSORT checklist（中文版）：http://www.consort-statement.org/downloads/translations
5. STROBE checklist：https://www.strobe-statement.org/checklists/
6. "中国临床试验注册中心"注册网站：http://www.chictr.org.cn/index.aspx
7. "国际临床试验注册中心"注册网站：ClinicalTrials.gov
8. PROSPERO（系统综述）注册网站：https://www.crd.york.ac.uk/PROSPERO/
9. PRISMA Flow Diagram（流程图）：http://www.prisma-statement.org/PRISMAStatement/FlowDiagram
10. Cochrane 偏倚评估工具：https://methods.cochrane.org/bias/resources
11. Joanna Briggs Institute 偏倚评估工具：https://joannabriggs.org/critical-appraisal-tools
12. Publication Manual of the American Psychological Association（第 7 版）电子资源：https://apastyle.apa.org/
13. APA 格式论文汇报指南：https://apastyle.apa.org/jars
14. CrediT 作者贡献详细介绍：https://www.elsevier.com/authors/journal-authors/policies-and-ethics/credit-author-statement

15. ICMJE 作者定义：http：//www. icmje. org/recommendations/browse/roles-and-responsibilities/defining-the-role-of-authors-and-contributors. html

16. Retraction Watch(撤稿监控网站)：https：//retractionwatch. com/

17. Conflict of interest form(利益冲突表格)：http：//icmje. org/conflicts-of-interest/